T0286142

For centuries so-called 'difficult women' have been labelled as 'hysterical' and 'out of their minds'. Today they wait longer for health diagnoses, often being told it's 'all in their heads'. Although health care systems are overburdened, why are women the first to feel the effects of this? Why is it so hard for women to find the kind of help they need? Why is no one listening to them? And why have so many lost faith in mental health care?

Drawing on the lived experiences of women, alongside expert commentators, recent history, current events, and her own personal and professional experience, Dr Linda Gask explores women's mental health care today. In doing so she confronts her role as a psychiatrist, recalling experiences treating women and as a woman who has received mental health care, illustrating the dire need for more change, faster. Women can't all be out of their minds.

Linda Gask is Emerita Professor of Primary Care Psychiatry at the University of Manchester. Now retired, she has been the Royal College of Psychiatrists Presidential Lead for Primary Care and has written about her own experience of mental illness in two memoirs, *The Other Side of Silence* and *Finding True North*. A lifelong feminist, she has an international reputation in the fields of primary care mental health and doctor–patient communication and has been an advisor to the World Health Organisation.

'I have had the privilege of knowing Linda for over 30 years and have always been in awe of her intelligence and incisiveness. I have learned so much from her and owe much to her. This book is testament to Linda's ability to distil complex ideas to narrative that will be appealing to a range of audiences. Linda spoke to an incredible range of women in writing this book – and gives voice to their ideas, experiences and concerns. That Linda also shares her own experiences is powerful and makes for an intimate read. The book is thought-provoking and should be recommended reading for anyone working in health and social care. Linda's call for social justice is well made.'

Carolyn Chew-Graham, OBE, GP Principal in Manchester and Professor of General Practice Research at Keele University

'A psychiatrist's clear, accessible feminist narrative of the mental health problems girls and women still face from childhood through to old age, pressured to care for others while not receiving proper care from the mental health system themselves. It reminded me of so many of the reasons why a feminist perspective helps us understand and live our lives.'

Maggie Gee, author of *The Ice People*, *The White Family* and *The Red Children*

'An interesting and comprehensive look at the current state of play, rooted in such diverse research and commentary. I love that there's 'ordinary' women's voices sitting alongside medics and counsellors and literary references from bell hooks to Margaret Atwood.'

Harriet Griffey, author of *From Burnout to Balance* and *Write Every Day*

'As a second wave feminist and as a woman who has experienced mental health services from both sides (as a patient and a highly experienced mental health professional), Linda Gask brings a powerful and authentic voice to the vital discussion of women's mental health. Thoroughly researched, yet highly readable, this book is shaped by the narratives of women who have a diverse range of experiences, arising from family, social, cultural, and biological factors. A recurring theme is how women are too often viewed as both 'too much' and 'not enough' making the task of expressing our needs a challenge that directly impacts on our mental health. Even the most marginalised women will find themselves in these pages, and will feel strengthened and validated by Gask's compassionate and first hand perspective. This book is a giant step forward in de-stigmatising women's mental health issues and is essential reading for anyone interested in the range of historical and current power imbalances in mental health.'

Annie Hickox, Ph.D., Clinical Psychologist

'Using the voices and experiences of women globally, and a broad variety of fiction and non-fiction, Professor Linda Gask guides us through the many subjects facing women and girls today, showing us where feminism has failed us by getting 'stuck' on single-issue divisive topics. Instead, Gask asks for a much wider approach – one that requires more listening, knowledge and understanding.'

R.F. Hunt, author of *The Single Feather*

'A really important book. Essential reading for mothers of daughters.'

Melanie Reid, *The Times*

'In *Out of Her Mind*, Linda Gask claims that care 'must always begin with listening to the patient or client's story'. And that is exactly what she does in this book: she listens carefully to stories told by women – of oppression, abuse, neglect, mental illness – recovering narratives that otherwise have been silenced, voices that have been ignored. This is a vital, informed and wise book that is alive to the challenges of 'feminist-informed' therapy and the failures of our contemporary mental health system, while also providing possible solutions, ways out of the current impasse. Above all, it succeeds in treating its subjects and subject matter 'with respect, kindness and compassion'.'

Jonathan Taylor, Ph.D., author of *Laughter, Literature, Violence, 1840–1930*

OUT OF HER MIND

How We Are Failing Women's Mental Health and What Must Change

DR LINDA GASK

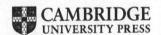

CAMBRIDGE
UNIVERSITY PRESS

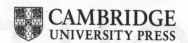

Shaftesbury Road, Cambridge CB2 8EA, United Kingdom

One Liberty Plaza, 20th Floor, New York, NY 10006, USA

477 Williamstown Road, Port Melbourne, VIC 3207, Australia

314–321, 3rd Floor, Plot 3, Splendor Forum, Jasola District Centre,
New Delhi – 110025, India

103 Penang Road, #05–06/07, Visioncrest Commercial, Singapore 238467

Cambridge University Press is part of Cambridge University Press & Assessment,
a department of the University of Cambridge.

We share the University's mission to contribute to society through the pursuit of
education, learning and research at the highest international levels of excellence.

www.cambridge.org
Information on this title: www.cambridge.org/9781009382465

DOI: 10.1017/9781009382441

First published 2024 (version 2, September 2024)

Printed in the United States of America by Books International, Virginia

A catalogue record for this publication is available from the British Library.

A Cataloging-in-Publication data record for this book is available from the Library
of Congress.

ISBN 978-1-009-38246-5 Hardback

For all the women

Contents

Contents

Introduction: Are We Out of Our Minds?

'Men are the losers now': Discuss.

Manchester 2016. An email arrived out of the blue asking if I would like to take part in a debate for Women's Week.

'Why me?'

'Because you know the facts – you are an academic.'

But I'm also a psychiatrist.

'OK, so which side do you want me to speak for?'

I didn't really want to argue for the motion but knew I *could* make a case for it if I had to. A good one. For two decades we have been bombarding men across the world to try to get them to talk about their feelings before it's too late. The suicide rate for men in the UK is three times the rate for women.[1] It has always been higher for men but since the crash in 2008 and the recession that followed, it hasn't just been young men who have been taking their own lives – the greatest rise for suicide is in middle-aged men who not only lose their self-esteem, but also sometimes their will to live when their jobs disappear and their relationships break down.[2] How we feel about ourselves and the way in which the world treats us has a significant impact on our mental health. It is key to our sense of wellbeing, and it can be very hard for men; but that's not the whole story. Many women are desperate too and women really *are* still losing out disproportionately, particularly in the mental health stakes.

'We have speakers for the motion', came the reply. 'We'd like you to second on the other side.'

Assuaging the slight dent to my ego at not being asked to lead with a huge dollop of relief that I wouldn't have to speak first, I agreed to do it.

Because women are still suffering with their mental health and are not being heard.

Gender plays a significant role in how we experience mental health problems. In childhood, the rates of emotional problems for boys and girls are remarkably similar but there is a rise in mental health concerns for girls in their late teens. Young girls seem to be harming themselves more often now than ever before.[3] The very process of growing up as a girl seems to have risks for the mind, and there is a widening gap between the mental health of young women and young men.[4] How much of this is to do with our biology, what we have experienced in childhood, the way we've lived our lives, or how we are treated?

During their adult years, one in five women in the UK, compared to one in eight men, experience a common mental health problem: anxiety and/or depression.[5] If you are a woman who is poor[6] and/or from an ethnic minority background[7] or LGBTQ+, you are also much more likely to have experienced these problems.

When men get depressed or anxious, they tend to be slower at seeking help because, as many have been told, 'big boys don't cry'.

That reluctance to seek help is something we try to challenge because of the higher suicide rate in men. But women's suffering may be at the very hands of men. This is not to say that women can't be violent, but, on average, a woman is killed by a man every three days in the UK.[8] Around a half of women who have mental health problems have experienced some form of abuse: physical, sexual or emotional. And over a third of women who have faced extensive physical and sexual violence in childhood and adulthood have attempted suicide. A fifth have self-harmed.[9] Women are twice as likely to experience post-traumatic stress disorder (PTSD) than men.[10] Why? Because sexual assault is a leading cause of PTSD and in Europe one in 20 women over the age of 15 has been raped.[11]

The ancient Greeks believed that madness in women was caused by their uterus (or *hystera*), a poisonous womb wandering around their bodies affecting different organs, including the brain. In the latter part of the nineteenth century, the diagnosis was made fashionable by Charcot, the French neurologist. Charcot's 'performances',[12] with their theatrical, misogynistic displays of a man gaining control over women through hypnosis, getting them to stamp on imaginary snakes, and even kiss the hospital chaplain to the audience's delight,[13] speak volumes to the fear that some men have always had of women's innate power and their desire to suppress it.

Society has never been kind to women who don't conform, and long before psychiatrists even existed and Charcot exhibited hypnotised hysterical performers in Paris, strange women who lived alone with cats as 'familiars' (I can put my hand up here) were likely to be thought of as witches and ostracised, or even burned at the stake. However, there is a long and well-documented feminist history of the troubled relationship between women and mental health services, and particularly with psychiatrists.[14] Haven't my tribe, the 'men in white coats', spent years oppressing women? Haven't we conspired, too, in ensuring women are likely to be described as 'crazy' or 'disordered' if they don't fit in? Yes, we have. I too *have* detained women in hospital against their will. However, I'm not going to defend psychiatry against the indefensible; and there is plenty for us to feel defensive about.

Over the centuries, many women, such as Mr Rochester's mad wife Bertha in the attic in *Jane Eyre*, and the eponymous 'Woman in White' of Wilkie Collins's novel, confined to an asylum by her husband with the connivance of doctors, have been locked away from the world. Sometimes this was for reasons of greed, because on marriage all of a wife's possessions, including her body, became the property of her husband; sometimes simply for being different, and wanting more freedom than society was prepared to allow them. You've only got to look at the records of admission to one of the old asylums to see some of the reasons given for why women were admitted, including exhaustion, overeducation, being unmarried or indulging in unconventional sexual impulses (such as masturbation) and even 'reading novels'. Asylums were clearly a useful solution for controlling 'difficult women' to get them out of the way.

But how much has really changed since then?

Like all the other women in the room that weekend in London in the mid 1980s, I had been drawn to listen to the author of *Fat is a Feminist Issue* who had inspired us to think differently about our bodies. The house was occupied by the Women's Therapy Centre, opened a decade before, by the author and psychotherapist Susie Orbach and New York social worker Luise Eichenbaum, who went on to found a sister organisation in North America. For the first day and a half the atmosphere was warm and companionable, until the moment when I revealed my profession. Then I felt the full force of a roomful of irate feminists towards doctors, and especially psychiatrists.

'What on earth are you doing here?' an angry woman shouted at me after I'd told her what I did for a living.

'We're the ones who have come to learn, to understand … ' I began, but my explanations were rebuffed. Another woman doctor who was also there to learn ways to help her female patients more effectively shared the outpouring of ire with me.

'You shouldn't be here,' someone said. 'We've suffered enough.'
But I stayed. Why? Because I was a woman too.

And a feminist.

What do *I* mean by feminism? Well, there has been a great deal written about the different *kinds* of feminism, but I think the definition by bell hooks is very clear: 'Simply put, feminism is a movement to end sexism, sexist exploitation, and oppression.'[15]

It's not about being anti-men. As hooks says, the problem is sexism. And the 'patriarchy' is institutionalised sexism.

Some feminist writers in the mental health field have argued that psychiatrists are the problem, when it comes to women's mental health, rather than the solution. Blaming women for harm caused by men by labelling them as 'mentally ill'. I have been told many times that giving someone a diagnosis is just a way of deflecting attention from what caused their distress and suffering in the first place, and only makes things worse, not better. I've been asked, 'Don't women just have more problems like depression and anxiety because their lives are harder, and they are oppressed by patriarchy? Wouldn't anyone going through what they suffered behave in the same way?'

These opposite ways of looking at the problem 'is it depression or oppression?' 'Is it madness or a sane reaction to an insane life?' will keep the argument going indefinitely. I believe mental illness *and* oppression both play a part throughout women's lives, and they aren't mutually exclusive.

In this book I will explain how *both* are important, and *both* are neglected.

The evening of the debate, in the green and white tiled hall of the People's Museum in Manchester, the audience were overwhelmingly white and female. That disappointed me. Women's Week is a feminist event, but if feminism is going to mean something, it must be relevant to those to whom it matters. Not just the women who were there that night, but to *all* women, regardless of their race, religion, age, class, ability, sexuality and whether or not they identify as cis or trans women. And some feminist writing has become increasingly opaque. No, unintelligible. I was very relieved when one of the people I interviewed early on for this book admitted to me that she, too, found some authors hard to read. I hadn't the guts to tell her that I found her own work almost as dense. The kind of stuff that, in her marvellous 'part memoir/part rant' *How to Be a Woman*, Caitlin Moran said was only discussed at 11pm on BBC4. Even though I'm an academic, trying to read it makes me want to rant too.

In a school debate, I had managed to be on the losing side when it came to the existence of God. Arguing with the fervour of a young scientist that there was no evidence for a 'higher power' up in the sky, I underestimated the power of faith in giving people hope, something which I always tried so hard to hold on to for my patients, the majority of whom were women. Trying to help them to believe that life was indeed worth living; that we could do something to make it more tolerable, even when things seemed very bleak. In some of the most deprived parts of Britain, such as South Yorkshire and latterly Salford, one in six of the entire population were prescribed antidepressants in 2017.[16] I also spent time trying to reach women from ethnic minority communities with mental health problems: the British Pakistani women of Levenshulme and the strictly Orthodox Jewish wives of North Manchester.

I didn't see any of them in the room.

'I guess I've spent quite a lot of my life working with women who would never manage to make it out here this evening,' I started off, realising there was still quite a lot of work to do to convince the audience. 'There are women who are not even able to come out on their own. Women for whom the idea of coming to a debate here, tonight, on this or any other subject would be completely alien. Women who feel embarrassed about being asked to speak out about their experiences. Women who live in constant fear of their partners.'

That evening I tried to speak up on behalf of those women. To remember why I had always called myself a feminist, even during dark days when the 'F' word became so unfashionable. To remember that there is so much more to do not only to improve the lives of women, but also to recall the tremendous enthusiasm and energy we had to improve mental health care for women, 50 years ago.

The leaders of the Women's Liberation Movement of the 1970s, the 'second wave of feminism', were fighting for equality (the first wave of feminism was about *getting the vote*). They had a great deal to say about what it was like to be growing up as a woman in a world run by men. And, as time went on, the close relationship between a woman's apparently less powerful place in the world (if she knew where she belonged, of course) and her mental health. They provided an explanation of how and why women, who across the world are subjected to pervasive sexism, harassment and violence, experience depression and anxiety at twice the rate of men. Why we are particularly susceptible to eating disorders. How from an early age our (sometimes complicated) relationships with our mothers and fathers play a part in how we feel about ourselves, the world beyond our families, and what opportunities lie ahead for us in the future. As a teenager, I didn't stop to wonder if I was a feminist. I wanted to be in control of my own life and, with a few hiccups along the way, pretty much achieved that, although sadly I failed to elude those common mental health problems (anxiety and depression) that women experience more than men.[17]

As I began to build my argument that night, my voice wavering with anxiety, I thought about how women are supposedly *irrational and unduly emotional*. There still seem to be some men who think it is our unfortunate possession of an 'out of control' uterus that makes us behave 'unreasonably'.

That *is* how we are viewed if we complain.

We are told we are 'out of our minds'.

I've been there too. For me, it can mean three different things.

Written off as merely 'crazy' anyway and wasting time. Simply driven to that point by the unfair ways in which we are treated. Or our reaction on discovering that our mental health problems are apparently less important.

Just because we are women.

Feminism was supposed to help us to challenge these kinds of attitudes in society and make life better, and happier for women. So why are so many women still struggling with their mental health? Did feminism fail? What went wrong?

Why is *still* no one listening and how can we make them hear?

Listening to women's stories, talking with my colleagues, interviewing experts in everything from feminist geography to forensic psychiatry and drawing on my own experience as a psychiatrist, a researcher and a patient, I set about trying to answer these questions.

This book is about what I discovered.

1

. . . . . .

Growing up a Girl

In 2021, Soma Sara, a 22-year-old Londoner, set up a new website to which harrowing testimonies, describing how girls and young women experienced a 'rape culture' in schools in the UK, flowed in at an extraordinary rate.[1]

There were accusations of sexual assault of girls as young as nine. Some claims reported shaming of girls after classmates had circulated intimate photos without their consent. Experiences of misogyny, frank sexism and sexual violence shook the establishment even more so because many of them came, at first, from young women at expensive, fee-paying schools. Their testimonies are backed up by the findings of the UK arm of an international charity: 58% of girls aged 14–21 report they have been publicly sexually harassed in their school, college or university grounds.[2]

Since then, Soma has appeared in the media worldwide, and everyone, everywhere is talking about 'Everyone's Invited'. When I was able to catch a call with her, she had just returned from rollerblading.

Suddenly I felt old.

I didn't burn my bra in 1970, when the feminist protesters famously stormed the Miss World competition in London, because I was still too pleased to be wearing one, but I was energised by the feeling that our moment, as girls and women, had finally come. We were not going to be ignored or patronised for having opinions, prevented any longer from doing technical drawing or woodwork at school, or playing football if we wanted to. We were going to be free to make our own choices in life, regardless of our gender. It was exhilarating.

Now Soma was telling me about the battles she was *still* fighting.

'What surprised me most,' she said 'was the scale and the speed in which it [Everyone's Invited] kind of took off and blew up ... we thought that it would take decades to give that kind of exposure to this problem. It was just an extraordinary tidal wave of voices.'

What these young women have begun to talk about is also closely related to our growing concerns about their mental health.

Tamsin Ford is the professor of child and adolescent psychiatry at Cambridge University, and she's been involved in a great deal of the research in this area in the last couple of decades. She is also someone I know personally. She possesses a warm and down to earth manner that I would appreciate if I were a teenager and needed to talk about my problems. Perhaps, I thought, she could help me to understand why growing up a girl doesn't seem any easier now than it did for me back then.

'So, what changes for girls now in their teenage years?' I started off, when we'd managed to establish a flaky Skype connection across the length of Britain.

'It's complicated,' she replied. In early childhood, boys with mental health problems *outnumber* girls, because boys are more likely to be diagnosed with autism spectrum, attention deficit hyperactivity disorder (ADHD) and behaviour problems. But then, later, it evens up. At secondary school age, emotional problems increase in both genders, but more so in girls. Then there is a *huge* leap, particularly in girls, in the 17- to 19-year-old age group with 31.6% of girls screening positive for a probable mental disorder compared with 15.4% of boys in the latest survey in England in 2023. Eating disorders were four times more common in young women aged 17–19 years (20.8%) than young men (5.1%).[3]

The Adult Mental Health Survey (APMS) happens every seven years in Britain, and thousands are interviewed. The last one, APMS 2014 published in 2016[4] concluded that 16- to 24-year-old women 'have emerged as a high-risk group, with high rates of CMD (common mental disorders – such as anxiety and depression), self-harm, post-traumatic stress disorder and bipolar disorder. The gap between young women and young men has increased.'[5] According to Tamsin, young women in their late teens in this country seem to have a significant problem with their mental health: 'Referrals to child and adolescent services have rocketed up and talking to colleagues on the front line it is nearly all young women.'

Young Women are Harming Themselves

Jane told me over the phone from London how her problems began during revision for A-levels, when she felt under pressure with her schoolwork, but there were also problems at home. Like many of the younger women I have listened to, her most difficult times were thankfully behind her, because the last thing I wanted to do in interviewing her was re-traumatise someone by listening and then being unable to offer any support.

'I started self-harming, and it ... kind of spiralled.' Her voice dropped and almost seemed to fade away.

'Did it help?' I asked.

'I was using it as a release . . . it helped in the moment, but I had to do it more and more to have that impact.' Often that is the case. She ended up in the emergency department of a local hospital and was then referred to Child and Adolescent Mental Health Services (CAMHS). Jane, who is Black British, was then in sixth form and not only struggling with school but also very worried about her family, who were going through a divorce. Her cousin, to whom she is close, had also been recently raped while away at university. The case went to court while Jane was sitting her exams and, not surprisingly, all of the stress affected her performance.

'It felt like a whirlwind at the time. I focused on my schoolwork, that was the only thing I had any sense of control over. That's what I blamed it all on. Everything else was just a bit too messy to get my head around.' It sounded to me like she had felt very frightened and powerless to change anything.

The methods people choose to harm themselves change with the times.[6] When I think back, I don't remember self-harm being a common thing young people I knew did when they felt stressed out, although I know it happened in my wider circle of friends and acquaintances, and usually when something traumatic happened, like the breakup of a relationship.

Like many others of my generation, I read Sylvia Plath's semi-autobiographical novel, *The Bell Jar*,[7] and identified with the frustration that the protagonist, Esther Greenwood, experienced with the limited opportunities open to her in life in American middle-class society in the 1950s as an intelligent, creative woman. A couple of decades later, many of us still felt, like Esther (and Sylvia herself), rigidly constrained by the need to conform to the expectations of others about how young women should behave. I never reached the point that she did, where she overdoses on her mother's sleeping pills and hopes to die, but there were moments in my earlier life when I considered it, feeling both entrapped by circumstances and hopeless about the future.

As a young doctor it was part of my everyday work to talk to people who had been admitted to hospital after taking an overdose of medication. Arriving on a ward in the morning there would usually be one or two young women, and they were more commonly women, hooked up to heart monitors because they had taken overdoses of tricyclic antidepressants, which can affect the rhythm with which your heart beats and be lethal in overdose. The effects of the other common pill that people overdosed with, paracetamol, can be counteracted if you receive a dose of an antidote within enough time at the hospital, and it is now much harder to buy in large quantities than it was in the past.

In the 1960s, overdose with aspirin was more common. That was the period when it became very clear to doctors that young women were more likely than men to try to harm themselves, but without the *intention* of taking their lives, usually because of difficult life events and problems in their relationships. A new word was even coined for it – 'parasuicide'.[8] Before that, until 1961, attempting suicide had been a criminal offence in the UK, and people did not seek help in fear of prosecution. A psychiatrist with whom I trained told me how he sent a distraught and sobbing girl (thankfully she was an actress) around six chemist shops in Edinburgh asking, 'May I have 200 aspirins, please?'.[9] No one refused, though she was asked 'Are you all right?' and told, 'You should go and have a cup of tea.' Everyone, but especially pharmacists, are more aware of the risks these days, though a cup of tea continues to be advice given to people in a crisis. If only more caffeine was the solution.

'I do wonder about the seriousness with which women's mental health problems are taken,' said Louis Appleby.

He's been one of the voices trying hard to get women's mental health problems on the agenda and was for several years the clinical director for mental health for the National Health Service (NHS) in England. We've known each other since we were students.

He acknowledged there is an issue, fundamentally, with how our society, and health services, fail to help women with mental health problems, particularly those who self-harm.

These young girls are viewed as 'wasting our time'.

They aren't seen as asking for help *in the right way* and not behaving like patients, and especially women patients, ought to behave. Doctors and nurses tend to reject people who expose their inadequacies. They feel challenged by people they don't understand and whom they are unsure how to help. They hope women will just shut up and go away, but it isn't clear how women have to behave to be taken *more* seriously.

In recent decades, self-injury by cutting or some other method has become increasingly common with a rise in the number of girls and young women admitted to hospital for this reason.[10]

In spring 2022, girls and young women aged 17–24 in the UK had the highest prevalence of probable mental health problems (31%) across all age groups of children and young people, and 71% of these girls and young women said they had tried to harm themselves at some point in their lives.[11] Young girls are beginning to self-harm at a younger age than boys[12] and girls from the poorest backgrounds are five times more likely to self-harm than those from higher income homes.[13]

The way in which young women are sometimes treated when they ask for help after self-harm is appalling. Lesley, who grew up in Scotland and developed an eating disorder in her teens, told me, 'I had cut my leg quite badly. The doctor just looked at me and stapled me up without anaesthetic and it was so painful. I don't think he would have done that if I hadn't self-harmed. Also, I don't think he would have done that to a guy.' Many young women who self-harm have told me this has been done to them.

Lesley reported to her consultant what happened, and the emergency doctor insisted to him that she had consented to it. She proffered a wry smile, 'You're always not believed.'

Listening to her, I had no doubt she was telling the truth, yet something like this encounter is repeated regularly in British hospitals.[14]

Why don't young women get believed? We've been trying to challenge such negative, judgemental attitudes for decades, yet so little has changed. It all seems to come back, once more, to women not behaving 'appropriately' and asking for help in the 'right' way. Louis told me about the rise in suicide in young women under 25, with the largest rise in suicide rates in 2021 since records began.[15] What is particularly worrying for me is these young women increasingly receive a diagnosis of 'personality disorder'.[16] That happened to Lesley even though she had already been diagnosed with an eating disorder. Fortunately, 'personality disorder' was removed by her consultant. Why is it so hard for women to get effective help? And should we even be saying someone has a 'disordered personality', especially when they are so young? There is often an assumption that self-harm is 'attention seeking' and 'a cry for help' but among those who self-harm the suicide rate is considerably higher.

Louis's own research team[17] found there were several pointers to the causes of why young people take their lives: experiencing abuse of all kinds, domestic violence, bullying, bereavement and the internet (including bullying on social media) and *these were more common in young women*.[18] He told me how he was worried about what he called 'normalisation of self-harm': 'It becomes a coping mechanism that society starts to sanction.'

In other words, it's becoming an acceptable and routine way of coping with stress. I don't know if that's true, but it's certainly something that more and more girls and young women are doing in response to what is going on in their lives.

For Jane, as for many young women, it was a combination of things, both schoolwork and a family crisis, that led to her self-harming. The perpetrator was a friend of her cousin, and Jane's uncle blamed his daughter, asking 'Why were you even alone with him?' When her cousin shared what had happened, it really affected Jane. She told me, 'It's a different culture, different generation, kind of thing but it's something we internalise. We have to be sure, because if something happens it will be your fault.'

Fortunately, she was able to get support from a therapist who helped her to recognise the impact of these pressures and to find other ways of coping with her painful feelings. When we talked, she described herself now as better, but still anxious. I could hear in her voice how deeply these events had affected her. *It will be your fault.* That's a terrible burden of responsibility to bear.

What else is contributing to the problems that young women are facing?

Social media and peer pressure both play a part.

What Part Does Social Media Play?

Social media can be toxic, but as a child psychiatrist, Tamsin insisted that the jury's still out on exactly what part it plays.

It certainly has its positives. Living alone for long periods during the Covid-19 pandemic, it's been an important connection for me with the world. There are several people who I first 'met' on social media only to connect with later in real life, Tamsin included. Young people *do* get help online, from WhatsApp discussions about homework to support from others when they are feeling low.

Starting college in India, Naina at first found Facebook a good way to connect with people, but after being trolled she withdrew.

'I just got scared of it. I would go to my classroom, and I would see people laughing, looking at me, and I would assume they were laughing about me.'

Later, she tried to return but told me how she would see other people having fun. Which led to comparison with her own life.

'And it left me feeling that I could be doing more, so much more. *Having fun'*.

Instagram and Snapchat seem to have a particularly negative impact on self-perception.[19]

Lara, who developed an intense phobia of food when they were 14, which then developed into anorexia, told me how they started documenting their journey on Instagram, and quickly picked up quite a few followers.

'I was the only person who was a healthy weight experiencing an eating disorder. And it really badly affected my body image.'

Constant comparison is a theme with so many young women.

'Everyone was trying to look as though they were recovering. And it seemed a very competitive world of people posting miniscule meals and body checks.

'It wasn't a healthy thing at all, for me to be there.'

Yet, Lara said, it still felt like a 'community' even though they recognised it was harmful. They did eventually manage to recover, but then relapsed later at university.

'By this point, I had around 10,000 followers. There were a lot of people who I felt were looking up to me. I'd let them down and I felt very guilty.'

The impact of social media seems to be greater on teenage girls than boys[20] and teenage girls are particularly more likely to be both bullied and cyberbullied. Those found in research to have an emotional disorder *did* report more hours online to researchers. It must be oppressive to see the world looking at you through the judgemental lens of Instagram.

Several girls told me how social media seemed to heighten and magnify the impact of what was already happening to them and how they seemed more preoccupied by what happened online than male friends and siblings.

Hannah, aged 17 and currently doing her A-levels, attends the same school as her twin sister Becky, in the south of England. She told me, 'Boys don't worry about just posting *whatever*. Girls, it's often a lot more, well not *staged*. But you could tell there's been five or six photos, and they've chosen the best one.'

As most research is just a snapshot of one point in time, we don't know if the problems people report with social media are causal or correlational. Are young women more troubled because they spend so much time online? Or is it simply that those who are feeling low or anxious retreat to an online existence? So, what happens online might simply be symptomatic of other difficulties.

The content of some sites is very harmful indeed. After the death of his daughter Molly, Ian Russell began to campaign for the media giants who control social media to take responsibility for the graphic content relating to suicide and self-harm that he discovered his daughter had been viewing on Facebook, Instagram and Pinterest prior to taking her life.[21] On these sites you could find yourself being 'coached' by a person or a group of people, posing to you as someone completely different, and meanwhile encouraging you to cause yourself significant harm. Even to kill yourself. On the notorious 'Pro-Ana' sites, some persuade young women with eating disorders to lose even more weight.[22]

Being bullied on social media is toxicity of a higher order than anything limited to real life, even though that can be bad enough. There is simply no escape from it. It *can* make things much worse, but this is a more complicated story than just about social media on its own.

It is about pressure, competition – and the requirement of young women to conform.

An Awful Sense of Pressure

Over and over, I heard the same word from young women.

Pressure.

Not only from others, family, school, peer groups, but also from what girls put themselves under in order to fit in and conform with what is expected of them. The burden of responsibility that Jane talked about was just one example. There were many others.

Lesley, who is now 30, and was diagnosed with anorexia in her teens, said that she hadn't thought much about the impact of gender at the time but had reflected on it when she was older. There were plenty of cues and so much pressure. 'Girls should be like . . . delicate, quiet, nice. Be nice. And don't be bossy. Don't be like . . . don't be big.'

She corrected herself. 'No one *says* "don't be big" but don't be *seen*. "Don't stand out." And yeah, I think that there's less of that pressure put on boys who are told "be leaders" and *are* told to stand out.'

Boys and girls are socialised in different ways. Lisa, a postgraduate student who grew up in a small town in Ireland, agreed: 'There's more pressure on girls from such a young age to kind of be like, neat and tidy and allow boys to be boisterous or be expressing themselves.' Girls get rewarded for being 'quiet and being proper'.

At Lisa's all-girls school the pressure to look and act in a certain way definitely contributed to her feeling bad about herself and her appearance. I could detect, even with our fragile internet connection, how deeply it had affected her. She told me there were unofficial 'rules' about the length of your skirt and the height of your socks that were understood among pupils, not imposed by the school yet subtly enforced by the other girls. These included the wearing of make-up, even though many girls weren't yet allowed to wear it by parents. 'At the time,' she explained, 'I'd be down on myself. I think if I'd had more self-esteem to fall back on, it would have been a great protective factor. I'm shocked how low my self-worth was.'

Bullying is a risk for both boys and girls. However, for girls, bullying is less physical and more about relationships: spreading rumours, nasty gossip and shutting people out of 'in' groups. So, it's harder to identify.

Hannah, still at school in England and doing her A-levels, said that girls tend to have an immediate ring of friends, and there is always an exclusive 'cool entourage'. She belonged to a group of quiet introverts that didn't really talk to anyone else. Characters in the films *Clueless* and *Mean Girls* came to mind. She laughed, 'No one watches those films and says, that is what my high school career is going to look like. You know that it's fiction. But at the same time, if I look at the people who I consider more vulnerable, they're striving for that kind of ideal, which is a little disturbing.' As ever, it's those who don't fit in and are struggling, whatever their gender, who are most at risk from being bullied, and cyberbullied, too.

It can have a lasting impact on your life. Recently, a friend of mine was moved to tears recalling how she was bullied about 30 years ago, mostly but not exclusively by boys, about her shape and appearance. I was bullied at secondary school for working hard. There was a clique of three girls, very much that 'cool crowd' who on one occasion placed a damp apple core inside the pages of an exercise book that contained my hand-drawn and carefully coloured in map for geography homework. It was ruined. They made my life hell, taunting me in the playground and ensuring I was never chosen for teams. These are the experiences we never forget.

Girls are also given very *confusing* messages. Sometimes they are told they *should* stand out, because that's how they will succeed, especially when they are in competition, not only with boys, but also with each other.

Lucy, who grew up in Lebanon but now lives in London, was very clear about the importance of standing out: 'You have to wear the cooler outfits if you are going to be thought attractive. I did feel that I had to be thought attractive.' I remember that too, and how hard it was on a limited budget when other girls with wealthier parents always wore the latest fashion and carried the best handbags.

However much feminism discourages competition between us, women *do* compete, especially when it comes to relationships – starting with being able to call someone your best friend. Something I'd forgotten about until sitting down to write. That awful feeling that the girl you thought was your 'bestie' has been seeing more of others and you feel left out. Even worse if they are all on a WhatsApp group that you aren't included in. Competition between women begins early and continues through our lives, even if as feminists we'd prefer to ignore it.

Then there are the problems that arise if you stand out in ways that a girl is not supposed to – by excelling at school, especially in science.

In co-ed schools it is still difficult to get girls to take up science, technology, engineering and mathematics (STEM) subjects even though they offer the best employment prospects. My attractiveness to the opposite sex in a mixed-sex school was considerably diminished by being more successful than them as one of the three girls at the time taking A-level physics and chemistry. However, it was very clear my physics teacher was more comfortable with teaching his subject to boys than girls when the 'lads' would all go along to after-school science activities he organised. Deciding to not conform, by not behaving 'like a girl should', can drain one's reservoir of self-esteem.

Naina, growing up in India, said she has always had to fight.

'When you are born your father has a question to answer. Should he save money for your wedding? Or should he save money for your education?'

She *was* given opportunities to study, but other family members were often critical of her parents for spending the money, and of her own choices too.

'I remember a relative telling me that you should not take this engineering branch, but you should take that one. Because girls don't do mechanical engineering.

'He knew nothing about engineering himself.'

Girls *can* do science and maths, but sadly so many still think that they shouldn't, can't, or don't want to.[23]

Lucy, growing up in an affluent home in Lebanon years later, still experienced that sense of being 'out of place' in maths. She felt patronised by her teacher when he felt the need to explain things to her in a class full of boys: 'He was a lovely teacher, don't get me wrong ... there were always more girls in the lower-class and I thought that's maybe where I belong.' It's tragic that girls still report how gender stereotypes hold them back at school.[24]

Despite this, girls are outdoing boys consistently in education and pushing themselves even harder. Expectations are powerful. Not only what people expect of you but also what you expect from yourself, or just don't believe you can achieve. Girls outnumber boys now in training for what used to be male-dominated professions, such as my own. Perhaps it isn't surprising that people are asking 'what is happening to the boys?' but that should not come at the expense of diminishing girls' hard-won achievements.

'I was told "you will have to work twice as hard as men",' Tamsin said.

Me too. My overwhelming teenage anxiety was about examinations. Getting through my A-levels, in which I did less well than had been expected of me, probably in part because of my state of near panic throughout. For Hannah, doing her A-levels in England today, much of the anxiety of her female peers is about preparing for what they are going to do when they have finished with school. Hannah was aiming high but told me of a talented friend with low self-esteem she was concerned about. She didn't want to try for Oxford, because she just didn't think she was good enough. Boys more often seem to have fewer doubts.[25]

And there is *still* a pressure to be in a romantic relationship.

Lisa experienced this at her school in Ireland, although she was convinced that would *never* happen to her. She began to become more severely unwell during her final examinations: 'I just couldn't really concentrate ... and I felt like I was going to ruin my whole future, and there was nothing I could do because I wasn't functioning.'

'I'll never, ever marry, I want my independence,' I told my parents, then spent an awful lot of time worrying about being in a relationship. That was the massive contradiction of my youth, and another reason why so many of us in our women's group years later talked so much about men. They let us down, but we still adored them or believed that we should.

I'm transported back to 17 again, sitting listening to my favourite album, waiting for the phone in the hallway to ring and trying to convince my parents that I'm doing my homework. Desperate to hear from someone who has promised to contact me when he comes back home, and he *is* home now. Of course, he doesn't call, and I can't call him, that isn't *done*, so I feel stupid to have believed he would. Broken-hearted, I avoided that music for ages afterwards. If my failure to hear from him had been publicly discussed on Instagram;

or pictures of him out with someone else had been posted and discussed; derogatory comments had been made about me by anyone on such a public forum or he had put up an embarrassing intimate photo of me, I would not just have been distraught. The shame might have sent me into a deep well of despair that I would have had problems climbing out of. The emotional fallout from broken relationships can be profound.

Today, some clearly manage to resist getting into a relationship in their early teens but, as Hannah put it neatly, 'There's kind of a pressure to hit the milestones and every single book on the shelf seems to be one of those trashy, girl meets boy, and they live happily ever after stories.'

Romance novels still sell in their millions.

I read them too.

Neither Hannah nor her twin sister Becky were in a relationship, and were clearly very comfortable with that, but many around them felt the pressure to find someone. Becky said she had overheard a person in her class getting very upset in the changing rooms because she had broken up with a boyfriend, not because she liked him, but because then she would be the only girl in her peer group without one.

That's tragic.

All this pressure to compare ourselves with others means we can push ourselves too hard – not only to meet our own high standards but also to seek approval from others. Perfectionism feeds into the awful repetitive thoughts about low self-worth that can trigger depression, anxiety, eating disorders, suicidal thoughts and dissatisfaction with how you feel about your appearance. All of which is more common in girls than boys.[26] It can affect every aspect of our lives. In our increasingly sexualised and glamorised society there seems to be more pressure on girls – to look perfect, *and* be financially independent, but to be able to run the house as well. So, a young woman must be everything.

But *only* within certain acceptable parameters.

There is one final pressure on girls: to 'stay safe'.

'Stay Safe'

Over half of girls and young women aged 11–21 say they don't feel safe when they're outside on their own.[27] Is it surprising? In England and Wales, the highest number of rapes within a 12-month period was recorded by police in the year ending September 2022: 70,633.[28]

Like Jane's cousin who was raped by a friend, so many girls and women have and still are being regularly subjected to sexual assault and even rape. That command to 'Stay safe' is something drilled into us from childhood. The stories posted on Everyone's Invited reveal the sheer extent and horror of the problem.

Thousands of women demonstrated on the streets of London following the murder of Sara Everard in 2021. She was walking home alone and stopped by a police officer, someone we are told to trust. We know from CCTV that he even showed her his warrant card. He then raped and murdered her.

Lucy, who grew up in Lebanon, was told by her mother, every time she went out, 'Don't go to the bathroom alone, always have your wits about you.' Her mother had given her safety rules that she knew by heart and are still engraved there to this day. 'I've always been hypervigilant … I'm always looking to see if there is anyone walking behind me.'

That is something we all do. Thinking about what we are wearing, what route we use at a particular time of day, what we take with us. I carried around my own personal weapon, a pointed umbrella, for years when I lived in a city.

Because I remember vividly being followed through the empty streets of Edinburgh when, drunk and more than a little miserable, I decided to leave a party at 2am and walk home. Terrified for a few minutes, and realising the man was now only a few steps behind me I ran and caught up with a couple going in the same direction, gasping, 'Can I walk with you please?' My pursuer laughed and turned around. So many of us have been there and can count among our family and friends, women who have been sexually assaulted.

For Jane, whose cousin was raped, fear of assault became a stark reality. That sense of responsibility, to behave 'properly' and *control* ourselves, is drilled into us, and we are held to account when we are blamed for how men *choose* to behave towards us.

As the founder of Everyone's Invited, Soma Sara told me, 'These are taboo topics, and when girls speak about them, they're often silenced, and invalidated and told that what they're saying isn't true.' Her voice dropped and I could tell that her passion was intensely personal, 'When I did try and stand up for myself, I was gaslighted,[29] and kind of ostracised a little bit by my peers, that's really powerful.'

Being silenced and disbelieved has a potent impact on how young women feel about themselves. It makes us doubt our own judgement and lose our confidence. We can feel humiliated, confused and despairing.

It's Not Just About 'Increasing Self-Esteem'

'She has low self-esteem, that's at the root of her problems', someone would say about a patient in my supervision group of young, female therapists when I worked in a psychological therapies service. Everyone else would nod, perhaps identifying, only too well, with the problems of the patient we were discussing. What was less clear was how we could increase a young woman's self-esteem in half a dozen sessions of therapy, which is all the health care system in England would allow.

Many women lack self-esteem, and we stock up on our reserves of it in different ways – by trying to boost how we feel about our appearance, performance at school, at work, and our success in relationships. Yet trying too hard can make us feel worse. Self-esteem plays a big part in our vulnerability to depression, our health, and how satisfied we are with our lives. You might expect that the wealthier and better educated we are, the higher our self-esteem should be, but there is little evidence of that,[30] and even though some of the young women

I'd listened to were from 'better-off' backgrounds, they were still seriously lacking it. We need to understand where all of that 'lack of self-esteem' in young women in our society originates, and challenge it at source, rather than only telling girls and women that they are short of it and must try to do something about it, all by themselves. Or telling them that they aren't resilient enough. It isn't just about what is going on inside of us, but what we, as girls and women, have to battle against in the world. For some of us the hills we must climb to feel good about ourselves seem like mountain ranges. We don't simply need 'self-esteem' but time and space, in conversation with trusted others, support groups or therapy, to deal with those painful feelings about what has happened to us.

Self-help, alone, certainly won't sort out that, and society isn't going to change in an instant either.

I love inspiring stories about women who have broken the mould of conformity that life tries to enforce on them, and who have managed to live their lives to the full – women who no longer worry all the time about 'controlling themselves'. I found it difficult to get into Glennon Doyle's *Untamed*, perhaps because I didn't personally identify with her story, but some of the young women I interviewed for this book all clearly did, and strongly recommend it. It is a powerful story of breaking free from having to conform with what other people expect of you. However, what concerns me more is the suggestion that we just need to buy something, read it, and that will solve our problems. It can just feel like the pressure to speak in the same kind of language about our lives, which inspirational authors use, is another kind of conformity. Has business just harnessed 'feeling good about yourself' to sell us even more stuff?

So where do we go from here?

What Must Change?

Attitudes towards women seem to have gone into reverse during my lifetime.

'My colleagues who are doing much more teaching say young men have just gone back to appalling ways of behaving, sexism and misogyny,' Tamsin told me.

This is exactly what the young women who post to Everyone's Invited are talking about. We are living through an extraordinary age of contrasting absolutes in which in one plane of existence the ex-president of the United States could boast about his misogynist views, and yet in another the #MeToo movement of the current fourth wave of feminism, a new eruption of consciousness, especially in the *online* world, is finally challenging the abusive behaviour, unwanted touching, harassment and frank assault that we women have always been told is 'just how men behave' when we dare to complain. However, alongside the rise of popular feminism, with its emphasis on body positivity, empowerment and building women's self-esteem has come the frightening rise in popular misogyny, occupying the same very public platforms on social media.

This behaviour is quietly tolerated in our society and is harming our young women. It isn't enough for our feminism for be popular on social media and to be, as Sarah Bannet-Weiser in her quite brilliant book, *Empowered*, puts it, 'all the rage'. Everyone's Invited has powerfully amplified the voices of young women and brought into sharp focus what they suffer in our society. From being unheard to being, at least, acknowledged.

Now we need to follow their example. Get out there and challenge the sexist structures in our society.

But not just tweet about it, do something.

There are some things we can lobby our politicians about.

They must get serious about the real damage that is being done to young women in some places on social media. At last, there seems to be some movement on this in the UK when it comes to sites promoting self-harm.[31]

Fast access to therapy is *crucial* for young people.[32] Young women have taken their lives when they have heard how long the waiting list for therapy will be. Every day is so important when you are young and what seems inconsequential to adults can feel immense because your experience of being alive is so much shorter. Therapy might also need to be longer than a few sessions only and provided more than once. Tamsin said, 'We don't say Ventolin doesn't work if you have another asthma attack.' We keep on using it.

Parents can get involved too both in lobbying politicians and in challenging providers directly to get those who are educating their children to do more.

Problematic misogynist attitudes to women and the key issue of 'what is consent?' needs to be addressed *head on* in sex education in schools and by the governing authorities of colleges and universities.

There's also a great deal that schools could do about bullying.

It has long-term health consequences and young girls should not be left to deal with it on their own or have to move away to another school, as my friend had to, to escape her bullies. Girls are much more likely to experience indirect forms of bullying that are hard to specifically identify, and more difficult to address. Nevertheless, we know there are effective approaches that can help, such as empathy training, peer group interventions and restorative justice.[33]

Much more support is needed for teachers trying to help girls struggling at school – and even more so since the pandemic. Teachers don't need training to be therapists, but they do need to have a therapist or counsellor working alongside them to support them.

The content of the curriculum can be controversial, but it must include impact of conventional beauty standards spread by advertising and on social media platforms on body image, particularly for girls. Social media teaching should be provided by trainers who are nearer in age to students. Young people who can talk about social media in a more realistic way than older adults often do.

However, parents must also recognise that their children are being exposed to sex and pornography at a much younger age now, online. It may be an uncomfortable topic to talk about at home, but it cannot be ignored any longer. It's the reality of our time. We'll come back to this and the growing misogyny in society in a later chapter.

Some things, we as women and girls must, as ever, do for ourselves.

We must all become activists too, but in ways that feel comfortable for us.

In the 1970s and 1980s, many of us met in 'consciousness-raising groups' to talk about our lives and the connections between our feelings and our experiences of everyday sexism, long before that term was coined. Out of that came the realisation that 'the personal is political'.

Likewise, Soma Sara talked about regularly reaching out to other women.

'It's about creating a space for people to share, that's free of judgement, of shame of humiliation, that's about listening and empathy; also making sure survivors have access and are signposted to any help that they might want or need.'

What we do for *each other* is important. The personal is *still* political.

Jane's close friend helped her to start talking, and that might be all that is needed, but a therapist helped her to find coping mechanisms she hadn't previously possessed. She also writes, something I've found helpful throughout my life. Overall, she feels much better now: 'I know a lot more about myself. Now it's more of an anxiety issue, less of low mood.' I'm pleased for her, but angered by the pain that she, and her cousin, had to go through just to grow up as girls in this world.

The pressure for girls to conform to society's expectations of them remains as powerful in many ways as it was for my generation and that of Sylvia Plath's Esther Greenwood before me.

Not only are the problems that girls and young women experience with their mental health not taken seriously enough.

The difficulties they still face growing up in our society are also *completely underestimated.*

2

• • • • • •

Family Life

For 14 years, almost every aspect of Britney Spears's life was controlled by others.[1] Struggling with her mental health under the judgemental gaze of the world media, she was placed under a 'conservatorship', a court-appointed restriction of her freedom, more usually reserved for older people incapable of making decisions for themselves, and often lasting for the *rest of a person's life*.

However, in 2021 Britney spoke out and the world listened.

She told a court how she had been forced to go on stage when sick with a fever, denied power over domestic matters such as redesigning her kitchen because her choices were too expensive[2] and, most shockingly of all, prevented from removing her own contraceptive coil. At the heart of this oppressive regime was her divorced father, Jamie, who as conservator was paid $16,000 a month from his daughter's multi-million dollar earnings in addition to a percentage of deals signed. More than Britney herself was receiving.[3]

As the #FreeBritney movement got underway, and outrage grew about how every aspect of Britney's life and behaviour which did not meet with her family's approval seemed to have been viewed through the lens of 'illness', she was finally set free from this extraordinary legal arrangement. It's difficult to imagine it ever being imposed on a male performer, never mind someone who still could go out on stage, day after day. And when she began to express her anger about how her father, mother and sister had treated her over those years, many girls, and women, who had quietly struggled to free themselves from the legacy and burden of their families, must have identified with her.

Families have the power to change the course of our lives for good or ill.

They have expectations, borne down across generations, of the particular and often narrowly defined roles that girls and women will play in marriage, child-rearing and work, and about what members can hope to receive emotionally, physically and financially from each other.

There is considerable potential for harm.

I spent only six months working in child psychiatry during my training, but that was long enough for me to recognise that some children labelled as 'problems' were not the problem at all. It was their parents. Given that it was up to Mum and Dad as to whether they continued to bring their son or daughter to us for help, if they didn't like what we had to say they just never came back.

Later I would meet many of the children of such homes when I worked with adults. Many still bore the emotional wounds of their childhood. Indeed, the psychiatrist R.D. Laing thought that the tight and often confusing emotional ties that bind us in the nuclear family could, of themselves, be a cause of severe mental illness; even something commonly called 'schizophrenia',[4] in which the person experiences strange 'abnormal' beliefs or delusions, and hallucinations as well as difficulty with thinking.

In the director Ken Loach's early film *Family Life*,[5] released in 1971, Janice is a rebellious 19-year-old who gets pregnant and, at a time when it was still considered deeply shameful to be an unmarried mother, she is forced to have an abortion. When she struggles to cope and begins to withdraw from life, losing touch with reality, her rigid and controlling parents, believing they are doing the best for her, arrange for her to be admitted to hospital. There she initially gets sympathetic and understanding care, clearly influenced by Laing's belief about the need to get to the root causes of her problem through talking therapy.

But later, under a different regime, she is committed and subjected to electro-convulsive therapy and forced drug treatment. In the final scene she is exhibited, passive and silent, in an echo of Charcot's lectures on hysteria, to a group of medical students. The conclusion we are asked to draw is that her behaviour is an understandable response to what she has experienced, and she is not 'mentally ill'.

'Difficult' behaviour by women *has* been pathologised[6] throughout history.

Women's behaviour continues to be judged against a different set of standards to that of men. Girls and women are still constrained within our society. Their behaviour can be *wrongly* viewed as a sign of mental illness. They can be told that they are 'hysterical' or 'out of their mind' when their emotional response is quite justified by what is happening to them. They are dismissed as 'crazy' when they are most definitely not. They are ignored and written off.

Their reality is denied.

But the pressures life brings us can cause extreme distress, and, yes, trigger something I *will* call mental illness.

'Illness' is a state of being unwell, physically, or mentally, which can have many causes and treatments, but is different from how a person would feel at other times. When I talk about *mental* illness, I mean something that *isn't* a proportional response to stressful life events and is more severe or is experienced quite differently. It affects our ability to function in the everyday world and sometimes just to survive.

Mental illness has multiple different causes, including *both* biology and what is happening in our lives. And just because I mention biology, it doesn't mean either that I think we need pills for all our ills.

Far from it.

To deny that a woman is experiencing a *mental* illness, and to suggest this is simply a 'normal' reaction to what is happening to her, is *also* a way of *denying her reality*. But calling this illness doesn't mean her stressful and traumatic life experiences don't matter. Of course, they do, very much, as they can act as the trigger for her becoming ill and prevent her from recovering.

Personally, I believe professionals should avoid giving an ill-informed opinion on Britney's mental health, although I'm sure that there are people who would hastily conclude that she, like Janice, is simply being 'labelled' as mentally ill by psychiatrists and her family. However, the pressure that people experience from their families can make the symptoms of mental illness worse, and sadly the presence of mental illness doesn't shield a person from society's judgement. Quite the opposite.

It stigmatises even more.

As a psychiatrist, one of my tasks was to try to make sense of exactly how a daughter's early complicated relationships with her mother, father and siblings had an impact on her mental health. To help her to disentangle those complicated family knots that Laing described so well even if I don't agree with him that they *cause* schizophrenia. These family knots can affect us lifelong.

Daughters

Our family is where we first learn who we are.

Parents teach us, in subtle and not so subtle ways, how someone of our sex and gender should behave. Girls get told what is unladylike – such as swearing and sitting with your legs apart. At home, and at school, in my generation we were taught how to sew, cook and clean. I took notes in domestic science lessons on how to wash the crockery correctly. Yes, really. I was not expected to go to university by my parents. Much has changed in the last 50 years but for many girls across the world some lessons are still the same. We are still held to a higher standard of 'good behaviour' and with that comes a predilection to feel intense shame.

Shame is a word that will keep coming up over and again in this book, because it's something women are almost programmed to feel. Shame is different from guilt. You can feel guilty for things that you have done, but shame is about how the world sees you and your own core sense of self-worth.

Lucy, who grew up in Lebanon, told me how, when she lived at home, she was aware of the differences between what was expected of her and her brother, who was a couple of years older than her. She would have fights with her mother over laundry (something so familiar to me), with her mother telling her 'I do a lot more than you do.' But she would *never* ask Lucy's brother to help. When he came back from university, her mother would say, 'He should be able to come home and have it done for him.'

'My brother is a better cook than I am. I never go into the kitchen, and I'm always made fun of. He *enjoys* cooking! But it's all "Oh boy, *he can cook.*"

I know it's kind of ridiculous really, but it did affect me.'

As girls, our parents also give us messages that we are better at communication and dealing with emotions, than boys.[7]

For Lucy, this became her responsibility within the family. When she was 17 her brother was diagnosed with mental illness. It was 'earth-shattering' for her mother because she felt very guilty that she had passed this on to him as it ran in her family. Lucy said, 'I felt like I had to mediate everything that was going on with my family because my father wasn't really understanding of the situation and my mom was emotionally wrecked. My brother had to try to figure out what the diagnosis meant for his future.'

Lucy became her family's 'emotional switchboard'. She couldn't ever imagine her brother being expected to play that role. 'I was happy to take it on when I was younger. But it just got too exhausting.' And it contributed to her having to go into therapy.

'I've always been the mouthpiece of everyone.'

Girls are more likely to receive supportiveness and emotional warmth from mothers. Through this, however, they are also schooled in putting others' needs before their own, which may ultimately undermine their own self-esteem.

Lucy felt pressured by her mother to take care of others in the family, both practically and emotionally.

'There are lots of things that aren't my responsibility that I've had to do. There was always pressure coming from my Mom.'

When her mother was away, she would return to her former childhood home, which took more than an hour, just to take care of her father: 'I just didn't want him to be sitting on his own.' She knew her mother expected this of her and felt a burden of responsibility to 'make everything perfect'.

She thinks this contributed to her later suffering from anxiety.

In the north of England, Jem also carried a great deal of caring responsibility in her family. Her mother has been ill for many years with an eating disorder and now diabetes. Since her parents split up when she was young, she has lived with her grandparents, and helped care for a disabled aunt. Now 21, she cares for her mother: 'It was doing what I'd always done, just more frequently.'

Jem has serious physical illness too, epilepsy, and gets very anxious and depressed. I could hear the stress in her voice as she told me how her mother had just been in hospital again for five weeks, and other members of her extended family were looking to her for support.

'They just said, "So now you can come in and help everyone else," and I was shopping for five or six people, but I was still having to go to the hospital and drop off clothes and medication for Mum.'

Whatever a mother's background, if there is family stress and breakdown, especially during her daughter's puberty and adolescence, this can affect a teenaged girl's mental and physical health.[8] And when families are struggling in adversity, it's girls who are more likely to suffer by getting anxious, depressed and self-harming.[9]

Living in poverty is hard. Poor housing, having limited access to education and fewer opportunities in life damage self-esteem and contribute to family breakdown, which then leads to even greater poverty for single parents.

Who, I found myself wondering as I listened to her speak, takes care of Jem?

She told me how she gets support from the women's group she usually attends weekly. She can be herself there, but the group stopped for a while during the first Covid-19 lockdown, which was hard for her. She now carves out some 'me-time', making jewellery, but when it comes to her future career, she is adamant that she wants control of her own life.

What does she want to do, I asked her?

'Something I choose myself. I've spent most of my life, so far, caring for other people in one way or another. It's not something I want to do in the future.'

Yet it is what so many women spend their lives doing.

Even though much *has* changed since my youth in Western liberal society, across the world many of these 'rules for living' *still* apply for girls and young women in their families. Families have expectations of daughters, sometimes subtle, sometimes overt, that mould us to behave in a particular way. To conform to a specific gender role, which, as Lucy and Jem describe, can be constraining and harmful.

I can remember how, in the 1970s during the second wave of feminism, the battle against this sexual stereotyping was fierce.

We believed that if we only tried hard enough, we could do anything we wanted. It was a time of extraordinary ambition.

However, my own mother had very limited expectations (and hopes) for what I would achieve in life. Getting married, living nearby and being available for shopping expeditions seemed enough for her. That was the expectation that her parents had of her in the previous generation.

Like Jem, I decided that wasn't for me. I pushed back and instead vowed I would get to university and escape from my family, both geographically and financially.

Like many other women, I also learned in my youth that anger was an unacceptable emotion for a girl, which might result in a slap or something harder, from my parents. So instead of shouting and screaming at the unfairness of the world, girls of my generation silenced ourselves. We experienced depression, guilt, shame and perhaps even turned to self-harm.[10]

Girls still do.

Susie Orbach was at the forefront of developing a feminist understanding of girls' relationships with their mothers and fathers and drew heavily on psychoanalytic thought: the way of understanding how our past experiences govern our present relationships that began with the work of Sigmund Freud.

Mothers didn't come out of this well.

However, for daughters who picked up and read *Outside In, Inside Out*[11] by Luise Eichenbaum and Susie Orbach, the insights, personal and professional, were quite devastating. Sometime in the past I underlined this paragraph in my own battered copy:

> Unconsciously mother gives the message to the daughter. 'Don't be emotionally dependent; don't expect the emotional care and attention you want; learn to stand on your own two feet emotionally. Don't expect too much independence; don't expect too much from a man; don't be too wild; don't expect a life too different from mine; learn to accommodate.'

The way our mothers feel about themselves, the difficulties they faced growing up, and the way they see themselves in us, their daughters, are all visible *in the way they behave towards us* – pushing us away and pulling us towards them at the same time. We struggle to separate from them because within each mother there is a 'hungry, needy, deprived, and angry little girl' whom we are driven, in turn, to take care of as we have been trained to do for others.

The toll of this criticism on mothers over the decades has been heavy with many blaming themselves, often unreasonably, for their daughter's problems (and being blamed by others too).

If second-wave feminism was hard on mothers, fathers were pretty much let off the hook. A father seemed to stand apart from that crucial relationship with mother and daughter, and many women have described to me over the years how distant their own father seemed. Some have noted how fathering can seem more like a 'hobby'.[12] In many cultures, fathers are still relatively uninvolved in bringing up their children. But father–daughter relationships can be complex. Reading the Virago anthology *Fathers, Reflections by Daughters*[13] in the 1980s, I discovered how my own need to please my father and never quite succeeding was shared by others too. The fear of failing a father, and going against his will, still exists powerfully for so many women.

Although mothers may play the major role in nurturing, fathers are crucial in helping girls bridge that gap between family life and work and relationships in the outside world.

They can make or break a daughter's confidence in herself.

Jem, struggling to take care of her mother and other family members, had continuing problems in her relationship with her father, who had remarried and had a new family. She told me how, instead of building her confidence by recognising everything she was doing for others, he undermined her too.

'I'd see him on the weekend, it would just be like two days of comments about how I looked, what I could do with my life and stuff.'

She can see now that this was more to do with his unhappiness with his own life, but at the time it hurt terribly. It must have felt very undermining.

Subtle power struggles also feature in many family stories.

I've realised that despite being a total autocratic patriarch in many ways, my father *never* made me feel that I would be less able because I was a girl. It's down to his confidence in me, not my mother, who would have preferred to control my life, that I was able to go out into the world and succeed.

But my own mother was certainly jealous of the closeness I had with my father as a child. She didn't like it that we seemed to find shared interests to talk about.

Daughters may also be envious of their parents' intimacy and feel shut out. Sometimes power shifts so that a daughter gangs up with their mother against father, sharing their anger towards him, and holding him in permanent disdain, or father and daughter against mother. An absentee father may be glorified by his daughter, while mother does all the hard work at home. Siblings and other family members too can make bids for control of power, especially if a father is absent or dies, as my own did when I was in my early twenties.

Even if men hold the power over their daughter's access to the world beyond home, women may fiercely guard their power within it.

Power

'Patriarchal bargaining' is what feminists call the strategies that women use to achieve more autonomy and security *within the boundaries* of their oppression,[14] and it can be cruel.

Kimberlé Crenshaw[15] pointed out that race, class, gender and other individual characteristics 'intersect' with one another and overlap. *Intersectionality* acknowledged that discrimination does not only occur because you are a woman. In some communities, women must contend both with multiple degrees of disadvantage and with the resulting struggles for power in the family.

When 20-year-old Rabia came from Bangladesh to the UK to marry her British husband as had been agreed by her own family, she had to join a new family where she was then repeatedly bullied by her sister-in-law, who was married to her husband's brother.

Rabia was distraught when her beloved grandmother, with whom she had been very close as a child, died soon after they were reunited when Rabia first came to Britain. She was desperately sad that she couldn't return to Bangladesh with her grandmother's body for the funeral. Immigration rules meant she wouldn't have been allowed to come back again.

Left alone with her new and unwelcoming family she was utterly bereft.

'All those people they were happy, enjoying their life, it didn't affect them, but it was a big gap for me.' She tried writing a diary. 'I explained my thoughts, what was going on inside me, I couldn't share my feelings with anyone.'

Her loneliness and sense of isolation was palpable.

She looked back fondly on her life at home where her upbringing had been poor, but close and loving. Now she felt completely on her own.

Problems eventually came to a head when she became pregnant and started to do less around the house. Her sister-in-law accused her of behaving like a 'princess'.

'My mum told me not to do any heavy work. My husband was helping me. That was a *big* issue.' This constant harassment from the other woman, who seemed jealous of Rabia's arrival and new status in the family, was like 'mental torture'. 'My husband was doing the heavy things, but I was cooking at the stove all day. What was the problem?' None of the men in the family got involved in the dispute. Later, Rabia's sister-in-law not only verbally abused her, but kicked her too. She began to feel very depressed and eventually tried to take her own life.

If young girls reach this point, it's not only the pressures of online bullying and exams that put them at risk, but the deeply painful even brutal things that can happen in families: bereavement, domestic violence and sexual abuse.[16]

Growing up with Domestic Violence

'No one talks about child survivors of domestic violence,' Mal, who is now 24 and identifies as non-binary, told me. 'We talk about child *witnesses*. But there's a difference between witnessing a crime as a completely detached onlooker and witnessing a crime as a child between your two primary caretakers isn't there?'

Mal's father raped their mother while she was pregnant with them. He had a history of violent crimes against women. He had a history of mental illness too, which made him highly unpredictable: 'One night Mum had to carry us out the house. Dad was having a manic episode and decided that he was going to fix the gas. We woke up to him sawing through the gas pipes.'

But that didn't explain or excuse his behaviour towards his family.

Mal didn't realise the impact all this had on them. When they were seen by a psychologist as a teenager, they didn't even include it in the timeline of Mal's life they constructed together.

'So many people knew that this was happening, but never called it trauma. To me, this was normal. This was fine.'

It wasn't until Mum said, 'Did you tell her about this time or that time? And the psychologist just kind of looked at me. And I was like, "oh, no, I didn't."'

In childhood we think, whatever pattern our lives take, 'this is how it is.'

Khatidja Chantler, professor of gender, equalities and communities from Manchester Metropolitan University, told me that if *repetition* of offences is taken into account, 'women are much more severely damaged and suffer the most serious consequences' from domestic violence.

But children are rarely asked about *their* experiences of being there too even if, as Khatidja has found in her own research, it was the child who called 999 for help for domestic violence in cases where their mother was eventually murdered. Afterwards boys are more likely to become violent and outwardly aggressive to others, while girls turn inward on themselves, get depressed and have unexplained physical symptoms.[17]

Kirstein Rummery, feminist and professor of social policy, grew up in a violent household with a father who was the product of a violent household himself. Domestic violence is often an intergenerational problem, and she is also convinced that her father had untreated mental illness. Kirstein pointed out the problems that feminism has in addressing the needs of *both* victims: mother and child.

'My mum was obviously a victim of domestic violence but didn't protect me and my sister. Her way of coping was to put us in harm's way, to deflect harm from herself. She'd sent me *into* the violent situations, particularly as I got older.

'How can I square this ... because my mum is supposed to look after me? But at the same time, she's obviously a victim. So, the *feminist* in me says, I have to excuse her, she can't possibly be guilty of things, because she was the victim. But at the same time, she chose not to leave or to protect her children. I see these dilemmas played out by social workers, who would call themselves feminists in practice, but then they come into these situations where children are at risk, and they *must* protect them.

'That's where some of the feminist ideas and practices get really, really difficult and confused.'

I understand that only too well from trying to support inconsolable women separated from their children, sometimes permanently, who were also themselves victims. There seems to be far too little attention paid to them. And courts are also often keen to allow fathers continued access even when both mothers and children are still at risk. There is a belief that *a* father, however bad, is better than *no* father.

Really?

The Best Kept Secret in the World

When a visiting psychiatrist from New Zealand presented his research findings from a survey of women carried out in Dunedin[18] to an audience at Manchester University in the late 1980s, many were surprised, even shocked.

He told us that 20% of women who said they had been exposed to sexual abuse as a child (estimated by his study at 10% of the sample of 1,516 out of 2,000 women who returned a questionnaire) were identified as having psychiatric disorders, mostly depression, compared with 6.3% of those who hadn't experienced childhood abuse.

I wasn't surprised or shocked because our awareness of the connection between abuse and mental health problems had been there, in the background but often unspoken, for a very long time.

This was simply the evidence.

In 1984, Virago published for the first time in the UK the first part of Maya Angelou's autobiography, *I Know Why the Caged Bird Sings*. It tells the story of her growing up in the American South and being raped at the age of 8 by her mother's boyfriend.

The impact and consequences are overwhelming.

Despite being found guilty, her attacker spends only a day in jail. Then he is murdered. This sequence of events leads the young Maya to become mute, for five years, fearing that by *speaking out* she had caused a man's death.

Angelou's fame, and her story, reached the other side of the Atlantic at a time when feminists were increasingly aware not only of the sheer *scale* of sexual abuse, but also of its impact on mental health.

About the same time Jeffrey Masson[19] caused a stir by claiming that Sigmund Freud, the psychoanalyst, had covered up evidence of sexual abuse in his patients who suffered from hysteria, which was then viewed as a medical complaint of mostly middle-class women with all kinds of physical symptoms that couldn't be medically explained. Eventually Freud decided that this 'seduction', as he chose to call abuse of young women by male relatives, wasn't real but 'fantasy'. That the women's desire to be seduced *rather than what happened to them*, was at the heart of the neurosis they were experiencing.

Florence Rush, a social worker and feminist, had written about this well before Masson, in 1980,[20] but as men's voices always carry more weight, she wasn't heard beyond the feminist community. Florence herself was abused in childhood and knew what it felt like to be 'gaslighted', to have the truth of her reality denied. She later held Freud responsible. By denying the significance of what he had been told by his patients, she thought he had encouraged society, and therapists in particular, to ignore women when they talked about being sexually abused.

Analysts have been arguing between themselves about this ever since.

However, Rush was right about the impact these ideas had on therapists and Western society.

Abuse *was* hushed up.

If the victim talked about it, she exposed her own supposed 'sexual motives' and shamed herself more than the offender. She was 'the temptress Eve', even for her therapist.

It was, said Rush, the best-kept secret in the world.

Jane Callaghan, professor and director of the Centre for Child Well-Being and Protection at Stirling University, explained to me how most abuse of girls and women takes place in the domestic sphere: 'Close relationships, family, friends . . . I think the evidence is very clear in that direction.'

Martina, who spent her early years in Eastern Europe in serious hardship, was bullied and physically and sexually abused between the ages of 6 and 16, not by her brother, or father but her older sister.

'I would be on the floor crying and she would put her foot on the back of my neck and tell me that if I didn't shut the fuck up, she would kill me', her voice quivered. 'There were times when she would put out cigarettes on me.' Her sister forced her to tell her parents that her injuries were caused by school bullies, even though she had to spend time in hospital.

It finally ceased when her sister, who had a history of causing serious trouble, was kicked out of the family home. But when it seemed she might be allowed to return home, Martina wanted to speak up but couldn't.

'I felt like I had this ball stuck in my throat. But I didn't want my youngest sister to have to go through it too. It was traumatising enough for me. I can't imagine what it would have done to her.'

It was her best friend and her friend's mother who eventually told her parents. Despite her mother's support, her father has steadfastly refused to believe her. She was forced to leave home too, and her relationship with him remains difficult.

Martina really wanted to make a point by recounting her story: 'When I tell people I was sexually abused. They automatically think it was by a man.' Women abuse girls and women too, and women abuse boys and men. Both are much less common, but they happen, because where *power* lies plays a big part in who is the abuser and who is abused. It's about power not sex, yet a witless social worker still had the temerity to ask if she had 'enjoyed' any of the things that had been done to her.

We do not know the full extent of child sexual abuse because it is so taboo, but the World Health Organization estimates that about 20% of women and 5–10% of men report being sexually abused as children, and every year about 150 million girls and 73 million boys under the age of 18 are raped or sexually assaulted.[21] Many go on to experience violence, deprivation and mental illness as adults too, *particularly* women.

But some have difficulty remembering exactly what happened to them.

Buried Memories

'When I was 12, I made my first suicide attempt. And the school found out and had to tell my parents.'

Fern's story differs from Martina's in that, for many years, she didn't fully remember what had happened to her.

'The story in my family was very much, "what you can portray to people is very important". So I never sort of thought "do I tell people what's going on?"'

She realised later, looking back, that she had functioned as the 'glue' that held her unhappy family together and that her parents relied too much on her emotionally, particularly her father: 'I was like, marriage counsellor . . . little wife. I loved him. I loved my mum. I knew these were sort of bad things. But I thought, probably they're bad, because I'm bad.'

It was during her first year at university, that she began to experience hallucinations. At first, she was given a diagnosis of schizophrenia. Later this was changed to 'borderline personality disorder', something that doesn't surprise but yet also saddens me. As does the fact that this home assessment, of a young woman who was by then an adult, was carried out in the presence of both of her parents, denying her any confidentiality.

But it was several years later, when her father, from whom she was then estranged, sent her a picture of herself as a small child, that her memories of abuse as *a child at that very moment in the past* returned to her.

'The bodily memories, the fullness of it. And I just remember thinking like that, I need to tell the psychiatrist about this; this seems very relevant now. I'm having flashbacks. I can't shower, I can't brush my teeth. I can't sleep. This feels important.'

Can traumatic memories be repressed and then recalled much later? Yes, they can. Of course, many people don't forget memories of abuse in the first place. Others just simply let those memories go because they didn't seem important at the time. But sometimes a trigger, like Fern's card from her father, can bring them back. Other people may realise, for the first time, during therapy that what they experienced *was* abuse, and then become very distressed. But memories 'recovered' during therapy may not necessarily be accurate. They may also be muddled or fragmented[22] and memories do weaken anyway with the passage of time.

Feminists observed how 'False Memory Syndrome'[23] emerged when we began to recognise more abuse in the 1980s and 1990s and there was a real backlash against both therapy and Feminism. Therapists, mostly female, were accused of invoking false memories of abuse, mostly in girls and women, by abusers, who were mostly men. As Sam Warner, a psychologist, notes in her book *Understanding the Effects of Child Sexual Abuse*, there are both incompetent or ideologically motivated therapists, and manipulative, self-serving abusers in this world.[24] And it hasn't gone unnoticed by the #MeToo movement that a world expert in false memories *chose* to be a witness for the defence of Harvey Weinstein and Ghislaine Maxwell, among others.[25]

But what we *cannot* deny is that child abuse happens, most commonly to girls, and its effects are long-lasting.

As Jane Callaghan said, 'Once it's happened, I think it's almost impossible to roll back from that and not be affected because it just shatters trust.

It shifts that sense that the home is a safe space.'

However, the relationship between trauma, abuse and 'mental illness' isn't a simple one.

There are undoubtedly many women for whom their mental health problems may be, as Jess Southgate from the campaigning organisation Agenda, put it to me, 'A legitimate and rational reaction to something traumatic that has happened to them.' The reality of what they have experienced must be acknowledged, not ignored or gaslighted.

But there are also feminists such as Jessica Taylor[26] (and in the past Bonnie Burstow[27]) who believe trauma is the cause of *everything* that is labelled by psychiatrists as 'mental illness' in women. For them, mental illness does not exist and *all* the mental health problems that women experience can be explained as an understandable response to trauma. They see psychiatry as merely a 'tool of the patriarchy' in labelling deviant women as 'ill'.

The difficulty with denying that 'mental illnesses' exists is that it prevents some women with more severe problems from receiving the specialist care they deserve – which may be their lifeline to recovery. And ignoring the complexity of their problems is just another form of gaslighting. Our society isn't paying these women sufficient attention *either*, as we'll see in the coming chapters.

There are some women with mental health problems who have no history of trauma, they haven't simply forgotten it, and a therapist who is constantly searching for trauma *can* cause more harm than good.

What Must Change?

There are no simple ways to prevent the abuse of girls and young women, but what worries so many of us is how little is done in our society to address the appalling consequences of it. Equally worrying is that, as Jess Southgate put it, 'It's disturbing how far girls have internalised messages of individual responsibility.' They believe that the whole problem lies with them and not with the society that has exposed them to so much abuse, poverty and violence.

Rabia told me just how long it had taken her to achieve a sense of self-worth, with considerable support from an organisation where women provide mutual support. She tells her story now to help others.

Sharing stories of what we have been through, and overcome, makes a difference.

Families who are struggling, whether with simply having enough money to survive, with structural problems in society such as racism and poor housing, or with difficult relationships, need help too.

That isn't simple either.

Fern's description of what happened to her brought back images of Janice in Loach's film. The difficult family problem solved when she was consigned to the asylum.

'My dad was just furious about this idea of family therapy. "There's no way you're going to pin this on me, like, *you're the mad one – that's working very well for us.*"'

Working with families *can* bring about change, but it requires people with the right skills and training (and support) to get families involved and build relationships.[28]

We must recognise and help young women who have experienced early trauma in their lives, which may even be at the hands of those supposedly there to help and support them. That includes not only families and guardians but also professionals and therapists, and other women too. There are many 'definitions' of 'trauma-informed care', and we will keep returning to the elements of it in the coming chapters.

What trauma-informed care *isn't*, as Jay Watts the writer and psychologist told me, is 'A two-day course that everyone has to do.'

She believes that much more thought has to be given, right from when professionals begin to train, about, 'How do we speak to people? How do we listen? How do we *bear pain*?'

And women's pain too often goes unheard or is dismissed – as either negligible or even *unbearable* to those who should listen, and so is ignored.

Fern was relieved no one pushed her to open up and speak about her father's abuse too soon, even though she feels sure her therapist suspected it: 'Because when I remembered, when I *fully* remembered, and I was ready to really admit to myself, I knew that those memories were mine. I knew that I was remembering something real.'

Getting access to the right kind of therapy *for her* was important, and that has included not only psychotherapy but also eye-movement desensitisation reprocessing, (EMDR) for post-traumatic stress to help her overcome the flashbacks she was having, and medication which has helped to stabilise her mood. She has a family history of bipolar disorder and has needed care for that too.

Jem and Martina have been able to move forwards in their lives with the help of counselling and therapy, which felt right for each of them, and which they were able to get easy and fast access to.

Martina's abuser may have been female rather than male, but this has not made her any less of a feminist. Discovering how many other girls in a group she joined had also experienced abuse and been told, like she had, that they were lying, and 'saying it for attention' made her angry. That continuation of the abuse by *total denial of their reality* is something so many young women have talked about with me.

So, how much do families really play a part in women's later mental health problems?

Having listened to adult women talk about their own life stories *and* talked about my own, decades later in therapy, when the events of the past still seemed as real and fresh as though they only happened yesterday, it is utterly impossible to believe that how we are 'brought up' doesn't affect our vulnerability to mental health problems sooner or later.

I realised through therapy, like many women, that I had to separate myself from a parent who continued to damage my ability to function as a successful woman in my own right.

Most families are not violent, or abusive, but *many* are struggling in an increasingly unequal world. The pressures and everyday traumas of our family life chip away at our confidence and self-esteem, fashion the lenses through which we will see ourselves, others and the world, and, perhaps most important of all, powerfully influencing our ability to make successful adult relationships.

Getting our governments to provide better material and psychological support to families is a mammoth task, something that is beyond what we can do as individuals.

But what is within our power, among our own friends, families, and communities, is to *do something* when we suspect that young women are experiencing trauma and abuse – to help and support them to find someone to share their stories with who is trustworthy and skilled; to validate and not ignore, minimise, undermine or deny the reality of a young woman's experiences.

Just three words.

If we share them and encourage others to try too, we *can* make a difference.

Listen.

Hear.

Believe.

3

• • • • • •

The Art of Starvation

From the very first paragraph of Melissa Broder's 2021 novel, *Milk Fed*, when her protagonist Rachel tells the reader that all that mattered was what she ate, when she ate and how she ate it, we know it's likely she has an eating disorder. At a time when there had been an explosion in eating disorders,[1] with record numbers of young people waiting for treatment in the UK since the Covid-19 pandemic,[2] Broder, who has herself been diagnosed with anorexia in the past, captured the zeitgeist with a roller coaster book about food, sex and love. Rachel finally admits, after years of being unable to be thin enough, that she is now 'too thin'. On gaining weight, she struggles to maintain the status quo by spending hours every night cycling to nowhere. Her mental life becomes dominated by images of food, calorie counting and fantasies about the girl at the frozen yoghurt shop.

Forty years ago, singer Karen Carpenter's wholesome image and lifestyle were the antithesis of Rachel's chaotic present-day adventures yet, for at least a decade, she shared something important with her. An obsession with the art of starvation.

On the morning of 4 February 1983, a few weeks after a stay in hospital, where then 33-year-old Karen had put on 40 pounds, her mother discovered her body lying motionless on the floor of her walk-in wardrobe. The coroner recorded the cause of death as 'emetine cardiotoxicity': she had poisoned herself with medication she had been abusing to induce vomiting and avoid gaining more weight. This fatally damaged her heart.

But really it was the anorexia that killed her.[3]

Anorexia nervosa has a higher mortality rate than any other mental illness.[4] Men suffer too, but it is around three times more common in women[5] and three-quarters of deaths from anorexia are due to heart complications related to low weight.[6] Also, 1 in 5 die by suicide. Agnes Ayton, from the Royal College of Psychiatrists, has said 'people should not die of anorexia or any eating disorder'.[7] Yet they still are.[8] And, despite this, many people, including even doctors, politicians and journalists, sadly still believe anorexia is simply a lifestyle choice of young women who think it's cool to diet and starve themselves.

The reality is very different.

Why Anorexia Still Matters for Women

'We still get so fixated on this white, teenaged, emaciated girl. Eating disorders can present in all different body sizes, genders, races and backgrounds.'

Hope Virgo,[9] who is a well-known campaigner in the UK for those with eating disorders, was keen to emphasise to me that if they are only seen as a young, white woman's problem, men don't ask for help or come late when they are already severely ill, and people from ethnic minorities don't get recognised at all. Furthermore, Hope added, 'only 6% of people with an eating disorder are actually underweight'. Why is that?

Well, there are three major types of eating disorder. Anorexia nervosa was first described in the nineteenth century by William Gull, an English doctor, long before bulimia nervosa, which was only recognised in 1979[10] and is, famously, what Princess Diana suffered from. Binge eating disorder (BED) was then only added to *DSM-5*, the American psychiatric bible, in 2013. Taken altogether, these disorders are still two or three times more common in women.[11] Bulimia and BED can also both lead to death, but they aren't anywhere near as lethal as anorexia.

Bulimia and BED both involve eating great amounts of food, often in secret. The hallmark of bulimia is bingeing followed by 'compensatory behaviours': vomiting, purging and/or overexercising. People with bulimia may have normal weight. However, those with BED do not rely on these 'compensatory' behaviours. Being overweight may cause such extreme shame and low self-esteem that they cannot look in a mirror.

People with anorexia, on the other hand, have an intense fear of gaining weight and try to keep their weight as low as possible by not eating enough, exercising too much, or both. They may *still* have relatively normal weight when they seek help. Anna Conway Morris, a psychiatrist who helps children and young people with anorexia, told me about the 'string test': 'You put a string around yourself, but first you try to estimate how long it will be. Most of the girls here pull out this massive length of string.' They believe they are too big when they are already dangerously low in weight.

Some with anorexia develop bulimic symptoms and use compensatory behaviours to try to control weight. For example, Karen Carpenter had been inducing vomiting after eating to try not to gain weight. Others only ever 'restrict' and can adopt harsh dietary rules, such as extreme veganism or 'clean eating'. I remember several such women in the shared student kitchens of my youth and much later in my out-patient clinic. Painfully thin yet believing themselves to be overweight; living on a diet barely able to sustain even a sedentary lifestyle yet exercising constantly and cheerfully insistent that they were really 'absolutely fine'.

Hope Virgo rightly expressed concern about eating disorders among men. But in England and Wales in 2021 alone, there were an astounding 44 deaths from anorexia nervosa of whom *40* were women.[12] That means women represented 91% of deaths from anorexia. For females between 15 and 24 years old, the death rate for anorexia nervosa is 12 times higher than for all other causes of death.[13] So, while it is true that men may also experience anorexia, raising a concern that casting it as a 'women's problem' may deter men from seeking help, the fact is that women suffer and die from it disproportionately when compared with men.

Why?

The Feminist View

'Few women have bodies they can live in', Susie Orbach reminded me when we spoke. This must play a part in their susceptibility to eating disorders, surely?

Since long before social media existed, there has been a belief that women must prove themselves by their attractiveness and desirability. In recent years the beauty industry has exacerbated this, with a constant barrage of bodies with which to compare ourselves. Teenagers are constantly presented with airbrushed images that are unrealistic and unachievable. Instagram has a particular impact on how girls feel about their bodies, something its owners would prefer to hide.[14]

How eating disorders have spread across the world has certainly convinced anthropologists of the role that our Western culture plays in the development of eating disorders. When Ann Becker first visited Fiji in the early 1990s, she found that women of all ages were heavier than those of the same age in the West. In Fijian culture, eating disorders seemed to be unknown and fatness was preferred over thinness. On her return in 1998, she found that, with the arrival of

American television, many young women had started to diet as they were no longer happy with their bodies.[15]

I've dieted on and off all my life. Like many women, I have never been happy with my weight or shape. In a college campus survey in the USA, 91% of the women admitted to controlling their weight through dieting.[16] Susie's classic book *Fat is a Feminist Issue* was very influential in the 1970s in drawing the attention of feminism to eating disorders, and the politics of weight and appearance. In the feminist spotlight, the anorexic/bulimic became somehow symbolic of the challenges *all* women had to overcome; struggling against the strictures of society that measures our worth by our appearance. We wondered whether anorexia was something that had its roots in the consciousness of all women.[17] Feminist writers described self-starvation as a reaction to the way society views women,[18] and particularly how that operated within a family where girls were viewed as lesser beings than boys, of which there are still plenty. In becoming wafer thin and frail, the anorexic succeeded both in being both ultra-feminine *and* denying her sexuality. Refusal of food was a way to show just how strong she really was: being both rebellious and compliant at the same time. In theory then, according to some feminists, *all* women could be at risk from developing eating disorders given the circumstances in which they found themselves.

Anna, a child and adolescent psychiatrist, notes how when girls are valued *not* for what they do but what they look like, and there is a cultural focus on being fragile, and small – something she calls, 'toxic femininity' – this can lead to serious illness.

She said, 'In almost every girl's story there is an episode where they remember someone commenting on their weight, often around the time of puberty.'

Clothing is so connected to our appearance that clothes shopping can become complicated. Helen, a librarian from Wales who is now in her thirties, has suffered from anorexia for over a decade. She told me how, when she went shopping with her mother in her youth, before developing an eating disorder, clothes were categorised as 'good' or 'bad' depending on whether they made you look slimmer or fatter. This provided her younger self with powerful messages about what being a 'good girl' was all about: 'Femininity was seen as being smaller, taking up less space, being more reserved.'

And it has always been *so* acceptable to discuss women's bodies. Lesley, the young woman from Chapter 1, who self-harmed and who is now 30, has received treatment for anorexia since her teens. She said that when she first started to lose weight, 'Everyone cheered me on, saying, "You're getting healthy, and you're looking good, you're exercising more."' 'Looking good' meant getting thinner and smaller, in the guise of 'getting healthy and fitter'.

It saddens me that even now, 50 years after that infamous Miss World contest when feminists stormed the stage, our society still judges women by their appearance and body shape in beauty contests, whilst claiming that it's really about their 'personality'.

However, alongside *Fat is a Feminist Issue*, there is another book I remember vividly from about the time when Karen Carpenter died. It was a memoir, published in the UK by the feminist Virago Press, called *The Art of Starvation: Anorexia Observed* and I was riveted by it when I first began to work in psychotherapy with a young woman with anorexia. Sheila McLeod tells how, as a teenager, originally from the Hebrides, finding herself at a boarding school where she struggled to fit in, she became unable to live within her own body to the point of becoming anorexic.

So much of what she said then echoed in what young women treated for it now told me about their lives and how their illness developed:

> Anorexia provided me with the illusion that I was in control, not only of my body, and my own status in the community, but of that community itself and finally of the biological processes which others around me were powerless to influence. In short, I became convinced of my own omnipotence. The conviction started from my body and the discovery that no one could prevent me – if I were determined enough – from treating it as I wished. I had discovered an area of my life over which others had no control.[19]

The Need for Control

The overwhelming sense of your life being controlled by others to the point that *all* you feel and believe you have control over is the size and shape of your body and what you eat is a familiar theme when listening to the stories of women with anorexia.

'The two things she most valued in the world – her voice and her mother's love – were exclusively the property of her brother Richard.' Journalist Rob Hoerburger summed up Karen Carpenter's sense of powerlessness over her life: 'At least she would control the size of her own body.'[20]

Child and adolescent psychiatrist Anna explained, 'When young people feel stressed, or there are factors that they can't control, like a parent's marriage breaking up, or bullying at school, they can become over focused on eating and control.' To compare your appearance with your peers is quite a natural thing for teenagers to do, but some become really focused on this: 'A girl said to me the other day, I would love to get smaller and smaller and smaller and just disappear.'

The weight loss often comes with a giddy euphoric feeling. You've achieved something, and that can become quite addictive. Helen, a librarian from Wales, gained the respect of others, for her ability to diet: 'It was so nice to be good at something, I've always felt like a failure.' But she admitted to me she was also aware of a darker side to that sense of being in control. People started to worry about her as she began to appear more and more vulnerable and 'pathetic': 'The more unwell I became I realised that that was very effective at controlling other people. Why would you want to give that up?' Echoes there of the 'omnipotence' that MacLeod described.

Second-wave feminists focused on the family battle for control between mother and daughter.[21] Mothers were seen as 'enmeshed' or overinvolved, and desperate for daughters to eat while fathers remained distant and detached. However, in *The Art of Starvation*,

Sheila Macleod struggles with both her mother *and* her father. I suspect her book appealed to me because of my desire for liberation from a disapproving mother *and* the patriarchy. It was something I identified with in my patients.

Looking back, I'm aware that I helped some young women with anorexia to summon up the strength to escape from what were sometimes very unhappy families in which they felt trapped. But then I antagonised their anxious mothers even more in the process. My belief was that their daughters were adults who could choose what kind of life they wanted to lead, but they, in turn, were worried that leaving would mean upsetting their mother too much.

Was I entirely fair on families? It's difficult to know *now* whether parents' attempts at controlling their anorexic daughters' eating habits really come first or are the merely *understandable* result of the family's desperate attempts to get a young woman to eat.

It was in their attitudes to families that feminists got it *seriously* wrong according to Jane Morris, a psychiatrist and psychotherapist in Scotland. Jane is a lifelong feminist, of a similar vintage to me.

'Nearly all mothers, when they are faced with a life-threatening self-starvation in the family, are going to behave in a completely crazy way. They are going to mother their child in a way that actually wouldn't be appropriate for a normal healthy autonomous teenager.'

However, a controlling family and culture *do* sometimes play a part in anorexia. Bushra Nazir, one of my PhD students, researched anorexia in South Asian women and the role that culture plays in what's 'right' and what's 'wrong' behaviour for young women. Surprisingly, given what I said earlier about the role of Western culture in spreading a desire for 'thinness', it isn't girls from the most Western-influenced families who are more likely to develop anorexia and other eating disorders, but those from very traditional South Asian families in the UK. Here, their lives are rigidly controlled.[22] Bushra discovered a struggle between parents and children over freedom to live their lives like other British girls, with some leading double lives. There is no word in Urdu, Punjabi or Hindi for eating disorders and young women with anorexia were a complete mystery to their families. 'She could start eating tomorrow,' one particularly angry mother said of her seriously ill daughter.

One of the young women with anorexia whom Bushra interviewed, a 21-year-old student still living at home with her family, ran away from home just after meeting with her for the first time, and was then admitted to hospital after cutting herself.

She contacted Bushra again later to tell her she wanted to finish telling her story. When they met for the second time, 'She'd taken off her hijab,' Bushra told me. 'She was dressed in Western clothing and completely different from how she was when we first met, when she was living with her family. She seemed happier.' Bushra was visibly moved by her memory of the changes in the young woman: 'That really got me.'

She had at last been able to gain some sense of self-determination.

But the question of 'control' and how it relates to family and culture is complicated. There are no simple answers. While these issues are often at play among young women with eating disorders, I've also met many women feeling oppressed by family and culture who *didn't* have a problem with eating. They struggled with something else such as depression, anxiety, or an addiction. To help, rather than just taking a 'liberate the woman' approach, we need to take a more individualised view. Think 'why *this* woman has developed *this* mental health problem in her life *right now*'. That requires a broader perspective on possible causes for anorexia in which biology also plays a part.

The Bigger Picture

'The research is definitely showing that it's 50 to 60% down to genetics.'

Hope's statement about the importance of inheritance and genes in anorexia was confirmed when I listened to Cynthia Bulik, a clinical psychologist who holds the first endowed professorship in eating disorders in the USA, lecture at the Royal College of Psychiatrists International Congress in 2021. I have always been uneasy about how useful biological research into mental illness actually is for helping people. The last few decades have seen a shift towards looking for biological causes and treatments. However, the genetics research is very convincing.[23] Our tendency to develop an eating disorder is, to a large degree, inherited, not simply learned from other family members. Eating disorders don't 'breed true' in families with the same type of problem, be it anorexia, bulimia or binge eating occurring in every generation. A scattering of the different types can be found throughout the family tree of a person who has an eating disorder.

However, genes influence our physiology.

Unlike most of us, people with anorexia feel most comfortable when they are in 'negative energy balance', that is, expending more calories than they are eating. They feel worse rather than better when they are nourished. Again, unlike most of us, they dislike fatty foods and find starvation tends to *relieve* feelings of anxiety, as they do not recognise hunger pangs. They are also much more active people naturally, and this may well be linked to their genes. They have a puzzling ability to maintain a low body mass index (BMI), and even after gaining weight, they lose it again and their BMI tends to settle at a lower point.[24]

Bulik says, 'Genes load the gun, but environment pulls the trigger.' Those triggers may be many different things such as abuse in childhood, bullying, getting involved in sports or ballet dancing where shape and weight get frequently commented on and, of course, dieting.

But anorexia isn't an inevitable consequence of dieting.

She also emphasised, parents are not to blame, but I would caution (as in Chapter 2) that unhealthy dynamics exist in many families, even the most loving ones.

It's worth saying here that diagnoses can change over time in one individual. That just demonstrates how imperfect they are for describing the complexity of our experiences.

Helen, from Wales, started off with bulimia, 'I just thought, "Oh this is a great way of dieting". I got some counselling, but it didn't really help. And then I started doing the ketogenic diet, which kind of kept me all right and kept me eating enough, but in some ways, it was a form of control. Then that gradually developed into anorexia.'

Were these different illnesses? I doubt it. They were just part of how Helen's particular problems developed over time. She also told me how she had anxiety, panic and depression as a child long before her eating disorder developed: 'I struggled going to school because of anxiety, but I didn't really know what it was.' People with eating disorders are also at risk of other mental health problems, which are closely connected with them.

Symptoms of obsessive compulsive disorder (OCD) are strongly related to feelings of the need to feel 'in control' that we explored earlier. OCD occurs when a person has repeated intrusive thoughts and/or feels compelled to carry out routines to cope with their anxiety. Some people might also be autistic, which can go unrecognised in young women (see Chapter 11). Lesley, the young woman who developed anorexia in her teens, told me in Chapter 1 about how she felt so desperate at times that she self-harmed too.

Jane Morris helped me to make sense of how genes and psychological factors, particularly obsessional symptoms with a need for control, can all come together at puberty, when anorexia often develops.

'The most obsessive people with eating disorder tend to present with anorexia and becoming gendered is a very, very disturbing thing.'

So, if you are an obsessional perfectionist, there's a risk you'll respond both to puberty and to the demands of adolescence with a huge effort to take control.

'But becoming gendered pushes you *out* of control. And I think that's true in whichever direction your gender is going, but if you find yourself falling into the female gender, it's probably more disturbing.'

'Why?' I asked, feeling a little foolish as I really knew the answer already.

It was never easy to grow up as a girl, but it's even harder now, and if you really value being in control, to have a body that appears to be becoming less powerful than the alternative is very challenging.

This doesn't include *all* young women who have symptoms of anorexia. Indeed, 40% only develop it in adulthood. But Morris says that it's those with a genetically hard-wired will of iron to get thin, and a terrible fear of losing control and living the life that others call 'well', who are most at risk of dying of starvation.

Less than 50% recover.[25]

What's Going Wrong with Treatment?

Several different things, beginning with using BMI as a marker for needing help.

Hope Virgo, who has herself recovered from anorexia, started the #DumpTheScales campaign because she wanted to challenge the idea that treatment for eating disorders had to be linked to BMI.

Stephen Anderson, a psychiatrist who treats adults with eating disorders, told me, 'Somebody with a BMI of 22 can be as psychologically unwell as somebody with a BMI of 12.' It makes no sense to link treatment to BMI and the idea of having to *lose more weight* to get into treatment astounds me, yet that is the reality of many current services in the UK.

Jenny, a 30-year-old nurse and therapist, told me how she asked for help, again, for anorexia when she was at a healthy weight. She knew she was deteriorating, but the service wouldn't even see her. At one point they said that her problem just then was something called 'Purging Disorder', simply because she was then only purging without binge eating beforehand. They couldn't offer anything to help with that. She didn't fit into a neat little diagnostic box, so she was turned away again.

'By the time I did end up going in as a patient, I was underweight.' Then her diagnosis was changed to anorexia, and she was told, 'You don't have to prove you are ill, you are one of our most urgent cases.'

That's wrong. She *did* have to prove it.

Similarly, Rachel Bannister's 15-year-old daughter, who developed an eating disorder after being bullied at school, was unable to be readmitted until she began to lose weight again.

'They said there were other patients who were higher priority.' In other words, lower weight.

As a result, her daughter just gave up, stopped eating and drinking completely, and thus needed an emergency admission through A&E. Only then did she become a 'high priority' for finding a specialist bed, but this was over 100 miles from home. Then followed an admission to a local general mental health ward, where Rachel was frustrated at the lack of understanding of eating disorders. When she tried to raise concerns about her daughter's lack of progress and her desperate need for specialist care, an attempt was made to label her as having a personality disorder. After a second opinion from a consultant at Great Ormond Street confirmed that the diagnosis was indeed anorexia, *and* going to the media, a bed was found, but in a private hospital 300 miles from their home with no support from the local trust for the family to get there or visit.

The recommended treatment for adolescents with anorexia is family-based therapy. It is impossible to provide at such a distance, but remote placements aren't uncommon.

'If you don't make a fuss, you get neglected,' Rachel said.

Rachel has been accused of 'exploiting' her daughter by talking to the media when I've absolutely no doubt that the struggle has, at times, been utterly devastating for both. Hearing her story made me even more aware of failing to hear what mothers were trying to tell me in the past. They have suffered, often through several generations, and may need their own help too.

Clearly there is a serious shortage of specialist care. Attending an eating disorders conference a few years ago, I noticed the exhibition wasn't full of drug companies as medical meetings usually are, but adverts for private hospitals, who are making a considerable amount of money out of providing care for (mostly) young women with anorexia nervosa. Some 60% of beds for eating disorder treatment are in the private sector in the UK, which would be a scandal if this was treatment for cancer. These places are run entirely for profit, don't provide desperately needed medical or nurse training in eating disorders or participate in research, which mostly takes place in university hospitals. It's a similar problem in the USA too, with most treatment provided away from university clinics[26] and medical insurance companies even debating whether to pay for residential treatment at all[27] as they are unconvinced about its worth. In the UK, private hospitals swallow up a huge amount of the budget available for treatment but don't give anything back.

In-patient beds are not the only problem. Jenny eventually had six months of day patient care, which was enormously beneficial, and meant she didn't have to go into hospital. However, only 30% of NHS Trusts in England have day patient places[28] and community eating disorders teams are seriously lacking too. Meanwhile, British doctors get remarkably little teaching about the subject (only two hours in 10–16 years of training)[29] so don't understand the need to get treatment early, even if we had enough specialists to provide it!

Treatment can be traumatic enough without all this hassle to obtain it. You are agreeing not only to gain weight, which is hard enough, but also to work at facing up to the thoughts and feelings that the anorexia helped you to avoid. It's not surprising that you might feel ambivalent. The best services, such as Jenny attended, work in partnership with the patient, using the latest evidence-based treatment, enhanced cognitive behaviour therapy (CBT-E) specifically for eating disorders.[30] This can be tailored exactly to what a person needs.

Agnes Ayton, a consultant psychiatrist and eating disorders specialist from Oxford, told me how CBT-E, which borrows ideas from several types of therapy, is very much about working in collaboration with the patient, paying specific attention to their individual factors. But what is needed to make it work well isn't *only* the skilled conversation between therapist and patient: coming to a shared understanding of the problems (the 'formulation diagram') and an agreement on what to work on changing, but also a transformation in the attitudes of the staff.

That's much harder to achieve.

'The idea that you are the *helper* rather than the *expert* is such an important shift in thinking for health professionals.

'There is this sort of pervasive idea that the staff are there to control the patient. This is reflected in the language "nursing observations". They are the experts, and the patient is the naughty child, not to be trusted.'

Many women have described this kind of experience to me.

Helen talked to me about her last hospital admission for anorexia.

'I didn't feel like I was treated as a patient but as somebody who needed to learn to *behave*. You're put on a "behaviour scheme", you know, it's like being in Borstal.

'I feel like it's traumatised me since I've come out of hospital. I have always felt ashamed. It's almost as if I was locked up because I can't behave myself.'

'Behaviour modification' in anorexia means you get rewarded for eating and gaining weight, perhaps by being allowed to leave the ward, or even have home leave, and punished for failing; for example, being confined to the ward and having additional high calorie food. It is still included in treatment programmes, but much more in some places than others, especially in Germany. In the past these regimes were much stricter and could even be brutal.

If anorexia becomes chronic, it can be much harder to treat. Then people get labelled as 'treatment resistant', and having a 'personality disorder', which becomes just another reason to say, 'we can't help you'.

The abhorrent idea that there is something called 'terminal anorexia', in which care should be withdrawn from the patient and they be allowed to die, has been ominously emerging in a world where effective care is being rationed because it's so hard to access.[31] People suffering from anorexia often don't believe they need help. And in this world, it's easy for anyone who isn't immediately willing to accept it to get pushed off the waiting list.

Personally, I loathe when someone is dismissed as 'not motivated to engage with care'. As a professional, my job was to work hard, using all the skills I had *to engage* my patient, so we could work *together*, as Agnes Ayton described, on a way forward.

This meant never giving up. And holding onto hope when my patient felt hopeless as many do.

Psychiatrist Stephen Anderson thinks we need to talk more about the trauma 'that is *actually caused by services*'.

I agree.

It's not just the struggle to get good treatment today, but also what some girls and women went through in the recent past.

We will return to their stories in a later chapter.

What Must Change?

Leading a 2021 review into the cost of eating disorders, Professor Gerome Breen from King's College, London, told the press: 'It's very hard to escape the conclusion that the fact that the disorders affect more women than men has influenced the level of clinical and research funding that they get.'[32]

That's a very polite way of putting it.

What this really means is that it is *way* beyond the time when all the things that have been promised should have been put into practice.[33] We need more treatment facilities, more research, shorter waiting times, better training of doctors, more joined up services, and for eating disorders to be taken seriously. We could do so much better in treating all the different types of eating disorder if there was much faster access to the range of treatments we already know can help.[34]

Services *must* change their approach. This would involve moving away from their reliance on BMI to decide who gets care, and only accepting those who fit into their rigid little diagnostic boxes; helping the person with the full range of other problems they have, not just their 'eating disorder'; treating young women and their parents with compassion and respect; working in collaboration with them; and taking the burden off mothers and getting fathers much more involved.

For some, existing treatments don't work. We need much more research to understand how to help them. Meanwhile those with long-standing anorexia need to know that they will not be rejected, but supported, encouraged and cared for throughout their lives. This just isn't there for so many women.

There are some things we can all do.

Remember that weight gain is normal at puberty.

Don't criticise!

Challenge our society's obsession with body image, treating us all, *regardless of our gender*, as sex objects, who must display our bodies to others, incessantly. This is the battle that feminism championed, but it's something the whole of society needs to get behind. It's damaging the lives of young people and eats away at the value they place on their true selves.

Nevertheless, I cannot help feeling that if there was less emphasis on how 'this problem affects everyone', and more focus on telling the *real stories* of different people struggling with eating disorders, however they identify, this would help us to understand exactly *how* the obsession with body shape and appearance affects us all in different ways.

Gender matters. Girls still suffer with anorexia more than boys. We cannot ignore it.

Finally, some will recoil in horror at the thought of treatments for severe, intractable anorexia that involve neurosurgery and deep brain stimulation techniques where electrodes are inserted into a part of the brain. It's a very controversial topic.[35] I remember the Scottish-Italian singer Lena Zavaroni, who died of pneumonia in a last-ditch attempt to avoid death from anorexia after neurosurgical treatment.[36] The feminism of my youth vehemently rejected medical explanations for anorexia, believing the cause to lie only in society's attitudes to women.

But it's much more complicated than that. Both play a part.

Feminism has not advanced sufficiently in how it thinks about anorexia. It needs to embrace the science that explains how some women are much more vulnerable to developing an eating disorder than others, and why biology also matters. This is something I'll return to again in later chapters.

Jane Morris, a psychotherapist by training, was suitably challenging: 'I'm a feminist to my roots but being feminist doesn't mean that you don't tinker with people's brains. Psychotherapy tinkers enormously with people's brains.'

Anorexia does too.

'On average, in Scotland,' Jane told me, 'Anybody who has ever been in hospital with anorexia has a life expectancy of 39 years.' Lena Zavaroni was only 35 when she died in 1999, just two years older than Karen Carpenter. That's not much progress.

Surely, we can do better than this?

Survival and recovery are possible, but it takes time.

Sheila MacLeod, the author of *The Art of Starvation* mentioned earlier in this chapter, did recover. She graduated from Oxford, went on to marry and divorce a 1960s pop star and became a writer. Like some of my patients, her problems with food, weight and shape persisted. Whenever she started losing weight, she found herself cooking elaborate meals of which she ate little or nothing and talking incessantly or dreaming about food. But she would eventually manage to start eating normally again.

She survived.

4

· · · · · ·

The Costs of Fertility

In 1892, Charlotte Perkins Gilman, an American writer and feminist, published a short story, 'The Yellow Wallpaper', about a woman confined to bed after the birth of her daughter. The woman was undergoing the 'rest cure',[1] a then highly recommended treatment for depression. Charlotte herself had experienced this, so she knew all about it. It was devised by a man, Silas Weir Mitchell, and prescribed that she be treated like a child, fed at regular intervals, and *never ever* allowed to sit at a desk and write again.

Instead, Charlotte sat at her desk and wrote an early feminist warning about the patriarchal role not only in controlling fertility, but also in managing the consequences of it.

In 'The Yellow Wallpaper', all decisions about the care of the woman confined to her bedroom are taken by her doctor husband. He believes he knows best and doesn't take her concerns seriously. Feeling increasingly helpless, she eventually loses touch with reality, and becomes desperate to help *another* woman whom she believes is trapped behind the hideous patterned yellow wallpaper in her room. There is no one else there. She has become *psychotic.*

Charlotte didn't become psychotically depressed but was very ill. She wrote how she 'came so near to the border line of utter mental ruin that I could see over'.[2] She sent a copy of her story to Silas Weir Mitchell, the great doctor who had nearly driven her mad with his 'rest cure'. Years later he admitted that he had altered his treatment after reading it (though of course he never thanked her personally).

Today many women do not choose motherhood. Half of women in England and Wales now remain childless by their 30th birthday, and mothers are getting older. The most common age for women born in 1975 to give birth was 31, compared with 22 for their mothers' generation born in 1949.

In her memoir *The Year of the Cat*, journalist and author Rhiannon Lucy Cosslett writes, during lockdown, about her longing for a baby, whilst acutely aware that she was still struggling to cope with the severe anxiety she has felt since being attacked in the street a few years before. Having spent childhood caring for her autistic brother, she questions whether she really *wants* to be a mother. Her perceptiveness about the way that motherhood divides and disempowers us brought back so many memories of my own friends lost to the 'other side'. By dividing us into those who do want children and those who don't, and by holding up those who 'decided too late' or 'changed their minds' as examples to ferment unease, patriarchy effortlessly manages to divide and conquer us.[3]

In my early teens I cared for younger brothers, one of whom had mental illness. I chose not to procreate. Some women are desperate to give birth but unable to. But many women, even today, feel they have no choice but to conceive and are still denied the *right to choose* by those who would limit access to abortion.

What we *all* share is the female anatomy and physiology that can result in both physical *and* mental health problems.

The costs of fertility.

Periods

There remains an extraordinary taboo and sense of bodily shame about periods.

They signify we have reached our potential to conceive, yet we must *hide* away any evidence of this. We live in fear of the blood stain that soaks through our clothes and is, horror of horrors, visible to all. Period poverty, where women don't even have access to safe and hygienic menstrual products, is a global issue. Imagine you are fleeing from an invading army, hungry, hot and tired and bleeding over everywhere into the bargain.

Becky, one of the twin sisters from Chapter 1, told me what she thought would help boys to understand what it is like to grow up as a girl.

'I'd make it compulsory for all boys to go through a simulation of the period when you learn about it in school.'

As someone who sat her physics A-level examination on the first day of her period and remains convinced that the dragging sensation in my pelvis, nausea, headache and fear of 'flooding' cost me a grade, I understood completely.

Pre-menstrual syndrome or PMS wasn't given a name until the early 1950s when Katharina Dalton, a GP in London, identified that her women patients had a variety of physical and psychological symptoms that coincided with their menstrual cycles.

Despite being the first to make the link between PMS and the female sex hormones oestrogen and progesterone, Dalton wasn't taken seriously by specialists in psychiatry *or* gynaecology when I was in training.[4]

In 1980, Sandie Craddock Smith was tried for the murder of a barmaid whom she had stabbed to death after an argument. She had a long history of impulsive acts of violence and self-harm, and had been in hospital many times, but when Dr Dalton was asked to examine her before the trial, she read Sandie's diary and discovered her violence erupted at intervals of 29 days. The prosecution accepted her plea of diminished responsibility caused by PMS, and she was given three years' probation for manslaughter.[5]

Whatever you think of Katharina Dalton, and her willingness to support the 'PMS defence' in law (with several cases that don't always stand up to closer scrutiny), she *did* change our understanding. And there *is* now good evidence that PMS is connected to hormones and is not only 'in the mind'.[6]

Sara, an Italian student living in London explained to me how PMS impacts her mental health: 'I get very moody, I cry a lot. I just get stressed.' Going on the contraceptive pill, made this even worse. The pill alone *can* cause depression.[7]

Pre-menstrual dysphoric disorder (PMDD), a more severe form of PMS, was very controversial for decades because women who are already low in mood can also feel much worse pre-menstrually, and antidepressants, particularly fluoxetine (Prozac), were heavily marketed for its treatment. PMDD was officially 'recognised' in 1999 but the rise of the 'PMS defence' had already led to anger among feminists who viewed all this 'hormonal' proof of women's unreasonableness as part of the conservative backlash against feminism. They asked, who might really benefit from the portrayal of women as unstable, inept and out of control during their periods? And concluded, 'It's a label that can be used by a sexist society that wants to believe many women go crazy once a month.'[8]

I know where these writers are coming from. Women *are* dismissed as *hormonal* just as much as they are called *hysterical*.

But is it fair to suggest we should just cope with it and stop complaining?

Those who experience severe symptoms and are desperate for help might beg to disagree.

Emily Grace has suffered with severe PMDD. She didn't respond to the usual treatments offered when she was diagnosed by her GP at the age of 26, confirmed after referral to a gynaecologist. She also had an eating disorder which she now thinks was simply a way of coping with her emotional turmoil. By then her life had, 'Just become like a mess of anorexia, overdoses and self-harm. This cycle that I couldn't get out of.' She eventually received treatment to block her menstrual cycle, along with the necessary replacement hormones, but was unable to tolerate any treatment with progesterone.

'Every time I took it, I basically went into complete crisis and meltdown, but just felt like I wasn't listened to.

'I went through lots of different treatments and struggled with being "compartmentalised".' Psychology would say, 'All your problems are psychological, there must be something that happened to you', searching in vain for a traumatic event in her past to explain her symptoms. 'Gynaecology would say "all your problems are hormone related".'

She was told she was intolerant to progesterone.

'I couldn't stand it. I didn't want to die. I just couldn't cope with what was going on anymore.'

Eventually a gynaecologist agreed to remove her uterus, fallopian tubes, ovaries and cervix. It's been a struggle and she is often very tired, having gone through a premature menopause, but is now able to work and live independently.

'Since that day I've not overdosed or self-harmed and have been able to achieve and maintain recovery from my eating disorder.'

Dr Hannah Short, a GP who specialises in both menopause and pre-menstrual disorders, told me that the causes of PMDD are complex.[9] There is a great deal we still don't understand, but perimenstrual problems are 'where menopause was, probably 10 years ago, I think people are just kind of waking up to the fact that it's a huge thing'.

Research into women's reproductive health is lacking. We *still* don't fully understand why women suffer from endometriosis, where tissue similar to the lining of the uterus, that bleeds when you have a period, is found in other places around the body. It can be completely debilitating, not only because of heavy painful periods, but abdominal pain, pain during sex and infertility. And then there are fibroids, large so-called 'benign'[10] growths in the wall of the uterus which are not cancerous, so don't get treated urgently, but can also cause debilitating, heavy, painful and prolonged periods in the endless time before menopause finally arrives (see Chapter 12). I've experienced them and witnessed the relentless psychological impact of chronic pelvic pain on women around me too.

It's very depressing.

We *still* don't do enough medical research into these problems to be able to help women's suffering. We don't really know how best to help them.

Now *that* is a feminist issue.

And there is still so much more to find out about the mental health complications of fertility, especially perinatal mental illness.

Perinatal Mental Illness

'Perinatal' is the period of time from when you become pregnant up to a year after giving birth. Ante-natal or pre-natal mean 'before birth' and post-natal or post-partum mean 'after birth'.

What isn't often realised is that up to 20% of expectant mothers actually experience depression and anxiety *during* their pregnancy and this then continues *after* childbirth.[11] It isn't *just* post-natal. If you are young, single, poor, deprived and struggling already with trauma or domestic violence you are more likely to experience it too.

Other women may feel quite well in themselves until after the birth.

Sally was 36 when her son was born. It had been an uneventful pregnancy and a natural childbirth with no complications. However, three days later she began to experience changes in mood, 'between depression and elation'. She was told this was probably the entirely normal 'baby blues'.[12]

It wasn't.

Returning home, she just felt unable to do anything to care for her baby, and everything had to be done by her husband and mother. She continued to struggle on, with support from her GP, who put her on antidepressants but she eventually came to the point where she couldn't cope any longer.

'I couldn't stop crying.'

When the psychiatrist she saw at the hospital suggested she could go home, she told him straight: 'If you don't do something now, I won't be here tomorrow.'

'I felt I was definitely suicidal.'

During her five months in hospital, she found it difficult to bond with her son, even though he was in a side room near her, converted into a nursery.

There was no specialist mother and baby unit and it felt like there was no safe space to learn to be with her son without interruption by other, often very unwell, patients.

Once, when there was a fire alarm, she left the ward on her own to go to the assembly place without even thinking about him at all.

'I remember feeling so guilty about that. *This was my baby*, and I really wanted him, but how could I not connect? How could I *not even remember* that I had a child?'

Sally's *only* treatment was medication, which she thinks only got her '50% better'. It was only after a relapse and a second admission that she finally received some talking therapy in the form of cognitive behaviour therapy, which she said did help her. She also gained support and confidence at a local group for mothers with post-natal depression.

She is quite adamant now that she did not get the 'right treatment', talking therapy, soon enough.

Trying to make sense of Sally's post-natal depression, it would be easy to point to her own past history of having been low when suffering from myalgic encephalomyelitis (ME or chronic fatigue), and her mother's history of depression too, as evidence of a biological cause. However, it's not difficult to see how psychological pressures (her ways of ruminating about her problems and worries) and social factors (things that had happened to her in her life) would make Sally vulnerable to post-natal depression too.

After talking things through in therapy, she realised how much her childhood relationships with her forceful mother and her brother, who was a drug addict, also played a part. She felt under pressure to be the 'good' child.

When her son arrived, 'All I could see was my brother, I couldn't see that he would be like his dad. And I kept thinking, "he's going to be like my brother".'

When Rabia (from Chapter 2), who came from Bangladesh to get married, delivered a healthy son, she had already experienced two painful miscarriages and her husband's relatives had continued to make her life difficult by criticising her 'untidiness' and even commenting on the colour of her son's skin, which was darker like her own rather than her husband's fairer complexion. She struggled to breast feed and felt increasingly hopeless, which was hardly surprising.

'I felt like I was *useless*. There was no point in living.'

After taking an overdose, Rabia was seen by a psychiatrist, and finally began to tell her husband just how bad things were for her. He began to stand up for her in the family home. That, and their first holiday away together, was the beginning of her recovery.

It's not difficult to understand how Rabia became depressed. There were no obvious biological causes, but possibly the sudden hormonal changes that happen after childbirth play a part in post-natal depression. *Possibly*.

We just don't really know.

Sufficient research *still* hasn't been done.

And why do some women become psychotic after childbirth, like the mother in 'The Yellow Wallpaper'?

One evening as a junior doctor, I was called to the maternity ward as the on-call psychiatrist.

A woman who had recently given birth had begun shouting and screaming, singing hymns at the top of her voice, and trying to pull a sink from the wall with her bare hands, despite the midwife and her partner pleading with her to stop. She seemed to have lost touch with reality and didn't believe she had a child at all. She was talking to God about it and said she could hear his voice speaking directly to her.

We couldn't hear his replies. She was hallucinating. We were concerned about her safety and the risk of her injuring or just exhausting herself. But she wouldn't listen. She had developed post-natal psychosis.

I've no doubt there will be some who will say that's quite an 'understandable' reaction after the pain and trauma of it all.

But is that *sufficient* to explain it?

Post-natal psychosis occurring within days or a couple of weeks of giving birth is thankfully rare,[13] occurring in one in a thousand births. But it can be a terrifying, dramatic change, from sanity to madness.

Sometimes post-natal mental illness takes the form of bipolar disorder, with episodes of mania or 'hypomania' and/or depression.

The mental health blogger known as @StrongestSmile on Twitter *did* have a difficult pregnancy.

'I never got to the glowing stage, I was sick about 30 times a day', she told me with a sad smile. Then, despite having an emergency caesarean section after 24 hours in labour, within a couple of days of returning home she was up ladders painting the walls.

'I decorated our entire flat. I held a dinner party every night for about three weeks!' Overactive and brimming with energy, with no need for sleep, she had become 'hypomanic' – a milder version of mania, but with no delusions or hallucinations. 'Because it was Christmas, I never saw the same midwife or health visitor twice, so nobody picked up that I wasn't myself.' And then when her daughter was five weeks old, 'Everything just fell apart and I dropped into a really deep depression.'

She struggled on for as long as she could, returning to work, but then, when on a business trip she told me: 'I was stood on the train platform. And you know when one of those trains come through the station that it's not stopping. It's going straight through and it's fast and it makes you almost kind of shudder. I remember thinking how easy it would be just to step in front of that.'

Terrified by her dark thoughts, she saw her GP urgently, and a few days later was admitted to a specialist mother and baby unit.

There, she tried to end her life: 'It didn't frighten me by that point, it was really well thought through. It felt like a rational choice, a rational decision to have made. Obviously in hindsight, it wasn't.'

She was discovered by staff just in time: 'I was so annoyed when they were putting that oxygen on my face. I just remember absolutely breaking my heart that I had to survive another day.'

Suicide is *still* the leading cause of death in new mothers in the first perinatal year.[14] In 2020, women were three times more likely to die from suicide in the year following childbirth than they were in 2017–19, and especially young and poorer women.[15]

Roch Cantwell, a gently spoken psychiatrist who has spent many years researching perinatal mental illness (and is a long way from the patriarchal doctor of 'The Yellow Wallpaper'), thinks beliefs and expectations about pregnancy and motherhood are key. For so many women the default position is: '"This child is 100%, my responsibility, and whatever I do, I'm never going to get it 100%, right"', which, of course, is true.'

But this interplay between extreme guilt and the sheer weight of responsibility of motherhood is crucial. It contributes to the familiar pattern of how severe post-natal depression can develop so rapidly, with both the profound guilt expressed by the mother and the estrangement at times between mother and child.

Roch told me that perinatal suicide has become *more* visible in the causes of death of women around childbirth, because death rates from other causes have fallen over the last century, although maternal mortality rates are still four times higher overall for Black women, and two times for Asian women.[16]

And despite being a wealthy country, the USA has the highest maternal mortality rate in the industrialised world due to a combination of racial inequality, high health care costs and lack of health insurance.[17]

StrongestSmile now has nothing but good things to say about the unit where she spent almost five months, eventually recovering after having medication, psychotherapy, and, more controversially for some (I'll return to it in depth later), electroconvulsive therapy or ECT.

'Without it, I can absolutely say hand on heart. I wouldn't be here.'

We don't understand what causes post-natal psychosis, Louise Howard, professor of women's mental health at the Institute of Psychiatry in London told me, but there certainly is a genetic component: 'In fact, there are some families where there seems to be a particular vulnerability to post-partum psychosis and *only* psychosis in the post-natal period.'

There is clearly a link with bipolar disorder, where a person's mood swings between deep depression and high, manic moods, with bursts of energy, overactivity and even delusions and hallucinations. StrongestSmile has a family history too, and since giving birth to her daughter, she has had episodes of both depression and mania.

She thinks that her traumatic pregnancy and childbirth triggered something which has proved to be much longer term. I think she is right, and that her genes also made her more vulnerable.

Not that we know exactly how.

However, there is also a feminist view that psychiatrists *completely underestimate* the part played by earlier traumatic life experiences in the onset of post-natal psychosis and therefore rely too much on drugs and ECT to treat it.[18]

I don't think it's a firm case of one or the other being the cause, because both biology and life events play a part. Our early experiences and genes make us vulnerable to mental illness, and both life events *and* physical stresses can trigger the beginning of it. We all try to make sense of our experiences and talking about what has happened to us is a crucial part of recovery.[19] But a person who is severely depressed can find it very hard, even impossible, to take part in therapy.

If you already have severe mental illness, such as bipolar disorder, you are at higher risk of having an episode after having a baby.

However, Louise Howard thinks too much talk about 'high risk' can be unhelpful: 'I try to emphasise the probability of staying well as well as the increase in risk of a relapse. Depending on the individual woman's circumstances it is usually more likely that she will stay well than not, and I am concerned that the terminology of "high risk" itself can lead to a lot of anxiety, poor sleep etc. which may be enough to cause a relapse.'

But how knowledge and information is shared, and understood, is key to making decisions. Not just about whether to get pregnant but also about what kind of birth you want to have.

Giving Birth Like a Feminist?

In *Give Birth Like a Feminist*,[20] the birth campaigner Milli Hill tells how women's bodies gradually became the business of men, and obstetric care became more medicalised, especially in the USA, where almost all care is led by obstetricians rather than midwives. She passionately argues for women to have more choice and control over what happens to them and describes birth as 'the land feminism forgot'.

It's clear that women *do* want a more positive experience of birth. Some women experience overmedicalised care – too much too soon, but others, especially in low-income countries, get too little too late.[21] Women's worries and concerns during pregnancy and childbirth may not be listened to.

Over the years I've met those so distressed by childbirth that they have had symptoms of post-traumatic stress disorder afterwards,[22] with flashbacks to what happened, a constant sense of fear and anxiety, and intrusive thoughts triggered by something that reminded them of the trauma of the birth.

For some feminists, childbirth rights have been more about being able to keep your career, work part time and keep up in a man's world, and less to do with what happens in the labour ward.

For others, even back in the 1980s when a member of the women's group I attended supported natural childbirth, at home, without medical intervention, feminism became *very much* concerned with the delivery and achieving a glorious, powerful earthy sense of 'real motherhood'. This was how women had always been 'supposed' to give birth.

Did 'natural' childbirth become 'feminist' childbirth?[23]

Rejecting the patriarchal medical control and taking back power, a strand of feminism moved from demeaning motherhood to glorying in it, even as evidence of women's superiority over men. Both natural childbirth and breast – rather than bottle-feeding began, for some, to assume almost a cult-like status which French feminist Elizabeth Badinter, criticised as making women feel guilty because they were unable to live up to the *perfect* ideal of motherhood. Even more to feel ashamed about. In her opinion, the baby had clearly become the best ally of male domination.[24] Meanwhile, in the USA, a conservative, Christian pro-family 'feminism' even began to emerge, with even more societal pressure.

Ruth-Ann Harpur, a clinical psychologist, who works with people for whom birth trauma has triggered issues in their relationship, told me about Grantly Dick-Read,[25] an obstetrician and first president of the National Childbirth Trust in the UK.

Dick-Read wasn't a feminist.

'He saw birth as being a kind of rite of passage, the pinnacle of womanhood and your femininity.' He was against middle-class women having pain relief, claiming that 'primitive' women didn't need it! I doubt they were ever asked.

Ruth said, 'Those ideas married up with those of people like Priscilla Briance, founder of the NCT who had lost a child after being harmed during labour.'

There's a powerful desire at work here of wanting to keep the white, male patriarchy of obstetrics and gynaecology at bay. Even though I've not given birth, I've experienced the, sometimes petty, indignities of gynaecology out-patients. Of being stripped of everything personal in the changing area before seeing the consultant wearing only a gaping gown. And I've also experienced not having my pain and discomfort after a gynaecological operation taken seriously.

Reading *Give Birth Like a Feminist*, I sense that medics are seen as more concerned about body than mind, and that the delivery of a healthy baby seems to trump all. But mothers, generally older now than in the past, are at higher risk of complicated pregnancies too. And birth can become rapidly traumatic when 'normal' delivery doesn't progress.

What happened to Marie during and after childbirth was devastating for both her physical and her mental health.

'I think I was coerced into having a vaginal birth.'

Marie was 37 when she gave birth to her son, after three rounds of IVF treatment. She planned a hospital delivery but received a letter saying they did not offer planned caesarean sections on request. This was a time, she realises now, when not only the NCT whose classes she attended, were campaigning for 'normal' or 'physiological' birth, along with midwives and other professional bodies in the UK, but hospitals, too, were trying to reduce their caesarean section rates.

Listening to her, as she told me about what happened, and the appalling aftermath, reduced me to tears. She was told everything about the delivery had been 'normal' but it was far from it. 'At the time I did not understand,' she said to me, 'But I *did* understand they saved my life.'

Following a forceps delivery, she experienced a severe post-partum haemorrhage. Then after the epidural anaesthetic wore off, terrible, unceasing pain. On returning home, in addition to the pain that was from her coccyx at the base of her spine, she had faecal incontinence, pelvic organ prolapse and also some loss of vision in one eye, for a few weeks, caused by high blood pressure. She couldn't sit down long enough to drive anywhere.

But nobody was listening. Everybody was telling her, 'This is just normal.'

Marie, feeling increasing distressed, blamed herself.

'This is who I am. I'm not a good mother.'

Her GP offered psychological therapy, but she said, 'I didn't want to talk to anyone anymore, they were not hearing me.' She asked for antidepressants instead.

Things got worse.

She shed tears as she spoke. 'I wanted to die. I wanted to kill my baby.' Tragically, this can happen when mothers become severely depressed or psychotic.[26]

Admitted to a mother and baby unit, the immediate concern of the psychiatrist was for her pain: 'So, you've had it now for three full months at level nine. And you don't have a pain management plan?'

Marie told the psychiatrist she couldn't understand how something that had been so traumatic for her was 'normal'.

To which the psychiatrist replied, 'But your birth was *exceptional*'.

Only then did Marie realise there had been nothing 'normal' about it at all.

Massive underfunding plays a significant part in why obstetric care is so inadequate in the UK – 'too little too late' obstetric care can happen in a high-income country too when resources are scarce.

But now, after investigations in several maternity units in England, including Shrewsbury, where there was overpromotion of natural childbirth, continuing friction in relationships between obstetricians and midwives and *even* blaming of mothers themselves for what happened, Marie's anger is palpable. The Ockenden report[27] found that 201 babies and nine mothers who died in Shrewsbury could have been saved with better care. There was a devastating impact on women under the care of the unit.

'Their babies died. This happened to me too, but on a much smaller scale. Stop keeping women in ignorance!'

Marie said to me that she wasn't provided with enough information to be able to judge for herself what *would* have been the best option for her delivery.

'I was told in the NCT class that spontaneous vaginal delivery was better for me and my baby. That's what I was told. So *why* would I want anything else?'

In throwing out the doctors and their 'male' science (even though there are more women gynaecologists now than ever) could women be failing to receive all the necessary information to make a truly informed choice? A choice based on medical evidence rather than natural birth ideology.

When a pregnancy *isn't* wanted, medical science is embraced.

But the right to choose, hard won by second-wave feminism in the 1970s, is now being taken away.

A Woman's Right to Choose?

In June 2022, the Supreme Court of the United States of America stunned the world by striking down *Roe vs Wade*, the 50-year-old judgement that gave women a right to abortion, passing the decision back to states to decide. Although state decisions are being challenged, abortion will likely become illegal in about half of the USA with, in some, no exception for *rape, incest or the mother's health*. Access to mifepristone, the medication used for early abortions is threatened. Even those who travel to other states can be prosecuted.

As reported by the *New York Times*, Dr Caitlin Bernard, a gynaecologist in the state of Indiana, paid a high price in 2022 for performing an abortion on a 10-year-old girl who travelled from Ohio.[28] Abortion had, at the time, been declared illegal after six weeks in the girl's home state. She has faced personal threats, prosecution and has been hounded by the conservative press.

When we spoke on Zoom from her consulting room, we didn't discuss the case. She was still waiting to undergo a review board hearing on her ability to practice and she looked exhausted. I asked her what impact limitation of access to abortion was having on her patients, and herself too.

> There's *fear* of getting pregnant, having an unplanned unintended pregnancy, or even having a pregnancy that is very well intended and planned. Having a complication, and not being able to get the care that you need.
>
> There's a lot of angst and pressure to use your contraceptive method perfectly.

There's also this feeling like you're living in a society that doesn't value you and doesn't care about your well-being. And is attacking women. I think this weighs on mental health. Something we hear a lot is that 'everyone is against us'.

Dr Bernard has experienced threats before. Many abortion providers have. Some have been murdered.

'It's taking years off my life.'

Most of the younger generation of gynaecologists in the USA are women. They are suffering too.

Dr Uta Landy is a veteran feminist who pioneered reproductive control for women in America.[29] Born in what was East Germany in 1945, her family escaped on a crowded train to the West when she was 10 years old, before the Berlin Wall was built. She has personally borne witness to the USA come full cycle on abortion. Prior to *Roe vs Wade*, hospital gynaecologists saw many with terrible complications of abortion, which convinced the medical profession to support it.

We talk about preventing access to abortion, but another way of putting it is that we're forcing women to have children. *It's forced childbirth*! Somehow, we are reluctant as a movement to embrace that concept. But I think that's what it is.

And the states where abortion is being prohibited is where the maternal mortality and morbidity are the highest.

This is especially true for poor and Black women.

'The effect on women in terms of their emotional response is very, desperate and very sad.'

The relationship between abortion and mental illness has a contested history.

Termination of pregnancy is neither a straightforward decision nor process, as Lucy Burns writes in her recent memoir *Larger Than an Orange*.[30] She is committed to being 'pro-choice' yet describes so vividly the confusion, regret and awful messiness of having an abortion. This, despite her unwavering belief that it is *what she wants*.

However, there is *no* evidence that having an abortion increases the risk of becoming mentally ill.[31] Indeed, some women have told me during my career how it saved their lives.

Instead, misinformation abounds, and women attending abortion clinics in both the USA and the UK are shouted at by protesters who stand outside waiting for them.

Alice, who had an abortion during her third year at university in Scotland, found the experience very intimidating and harassing.

'To go into an appointment feeling dissociated or a bit out of your head, because of the way these protests have made you feel is the last thing that you want when you have to speak to a health care professional and make what for many people is a big decision.' She was quite sure it was right for her, but it was still an awful experience. 'You know, we can't help but feel shame or maybe guilt around these issues.'

This is how we are taught to think from an early age. As a junior doctor I remember the 'walk of shame' that those coming into the gynae ward for abortion had to suffer as they went past all the other women, some suffering with infertility and miscarriage, to their separate room at the end.

Everyone knew why they were there.

Lucy Grieve, the cofounder of Back Off Scotland that has been campaigning for protest exclusion zones around clinics in Scotland, told me about one woman who, after attending a clinic for care following a miscarriage, experienced flashbacks after protestors accused her of murdering her unborn child. Doctors have had to try to keep patients inside calm, as amplified voices boom out.

'How is that allowed to go unchallenged?'

If this were happening to men, it would have been stopped by now.

Francesca Moore, a feminist geographer at the University of Cambridge told me: 'Much of the way that governments across the world are interested in *women* is about their reproductivity, and about all the regulations around things like abortion and access to health care.'

She is currently researching how American anti-abortion protestors are getting involved in the UK.

'When you interview protesters, they say, "Well, I'm articulating my first amendment rights here."'

Well, the American constitution doesn't apply to the UK.

But that doesn't mean we should take *our* rights for granted either.

Extreme American abortion 'abolitionists', antagonistic to abortion for *any* reason, are actively disseminating their ideology.[32] They seem to want to *punish* women for the transgression of seeking to control their own bodies.

Even for having sex in the first place.

This is terrifying. There will be an enormous toll on women's physical *and* mental health.

What Must Change?

Shame and *guilt* are words that come up so often when women are discussing the impact of fertility on their mental wellbeing, from menstruation to choices about childbirth and post-natal complications. There is the potential for great joy, but the costs are considerable too. Suffering is *real*, but women are still often not being believed or respected.

First of all, we should, as women, reject the artificial divide between those of us who do and don't have children and cherish those friendships. Coping with the lifelong complications of fertility can be a lonely place, *whether or not* you are a mother.

What we can *all* do is advocate and support fellow women who are struggling with any of the complications of fertility and not getting the care they need. Help them to find the care they need and to get referred to the right place. Go with them to see the doctor. Even write letters with them to their MP, and to the press.

Help each other to get things done.

When women's personal experience and energy is combined with social media savvy and solid support from a group of women health professionals, the media really starts to take notice. This happened with the Five X More campaign,[33] started by two committed young Black women in 2019 in London, who have massively raised the profile of the urgent need for better maternal health outcomes for Black women.

We should be learning from them.

There are 'red flags' we can all remember for getting mental health care involved in the perinatal period: a sudden change in mental state – how you are thinking and behaving. *Any* symptoms, thoughts or acts of violent self-harm to self or to the baby, thoughts about being incompetent as a mother or feeling distant and estranged from your child. *Any* self-harm during pregnancy or soon after birth is seriously worrying.

These are right there in the stories of Marie, StrongestSmile and Sally.

All professionals involved in perinatal care *must* be able to recognise these. Communication between them is crucial in keeping women alive.

There *are* many battles to fight against the patriarchy in ensuring that the complications of fertility get addressed, just not necessarily the ones that some feminist writers have identified.

There is a long list of things that feminists should be campaigning for: investment in women's services, obstetrics and gynaecology, which would not be in such a parlous state if they cared for men; better treatment for women with serious menstrual problems, not dismissing them; better care for women with persistent, awful, pelvic pain; better perinatal mental health care, not only for mothers, but also for the future wellbeing of their children[34] and the protection of abortion rights, which we should *never* assume are safe.

Providing pregnant women with the information to make truly informed decisions about their health care is crucial. Why can't some feminists embrace medical science and enable women not only to *choose* but also to *fully understand* that choice? And to be able to weigh up the evidence for the different approaches on offer, including alternative remedies. Are we *still* assuming that 'women don't get science'?

Some therapists still sadly search around for trauma in a woman's past history that may not exist, telling her that 'mental illness' isn't real, or that if she accepts medical or psychiatric care she is bowing to the medical patriarchy. Even though perinatal mental illness can kill. This does not help.

It's just *another kind* of gaslighting.

5

Women's Work

Just before Christmas 1965, 29-year-old Hannah Gavron, a mother of two who had recently finished her first book *The Captive Wife*,[1] based on her doctoral research, was found dead by a gas fitter in the flat of her friend in Primrose Hill, London.

The brilliant young researcher and writer had taken her own life.

Forty years later, one of her sons, the journalist Jeremy Gavron, wrote a compelling memoir of Hannah. Almost a detective story, it seeks to understand what happened in Hannah's life that would cause her to take such a fateful decision. Gavron called the story of his mother *A Woman on the Edge of Time*,[2] because, he said, 'this particular moment in history was in some ways toxic for this particular person'.[3]

At the time of Hannah's premature death, the impact of Betty Friedan's *The Feminine Mystique*[4] had not yet reached the UK.

Friedan, a former journalist turned 'homemaker', wrote eloquently about the discontent of women for whom their homes had become a prison, as society demanded they lose all hope of using their creative talents and become housewives and mothers.

In the years I've spent with women who were seriously depressed, I've learned just how much *emotional* and *physical* work women do in holding families together – mothering, problem-solving, labouring and coping in a world that undervalues women's work.

Betty Friedan called this 'ailment' that was causing women misery and despair, 'the problem with no name'.

The Problem with No Name

In the past, there's no doubt whatsoever that psychiatry's response to women who refused to comply with the accepted norms of femininity was brutal.

They were diagnosed with mental illness, sedated, given ECT and even operated on. In the USA of the 1940s, neurologists Walter Freeman and James Watts sometimes carried out 25 pre-frontal lobotomies a day, drilling into the brain and severing connections with the prefrontal cortex. A whole range of different diagnoses were used as justification: 'emotional tension, depression, obsession, compulsions, anxiety, hypochondriasis and psychosis'.[5]

In other words, anything you would care to mention.

As historian Elinor Cleghorn wrote about in *Unwell Women*, any kind of behaviour that didn't meet with the patriarchal view of the perfect wife[6] might be used as justification. And even though there were far more men institutionalised in the USA than women at the time, most patients lobotomised were women.[7]

One husband was even reported to have described his wife as 'more normal than she has ever been', afterwards. I am old enough to have met, in my early years as a consultant psychiatrist, people who had been lobotomised – blank-faced, passive and lacking in spontaneity. So that was 'normal'.

However, by the middle of the twentieth century there was another solution on the horizon to control difficult women suffering from the 'problem with no name'.

Tranquillisers.

At one time during my childhood, my late mother, whose unhappiness with her life manifested as severe anxiety, was taking two benzodiazepines at the same time – Valium (diazepam) and Ativan (lorazepam). I don't think her GP had intended that, but it wasn't questioned by the pharmacist dispensing it. Following in her footsteps, I too was prescribed a 'benzo' as a depressed and anxious medical student.

By 1968, Valium was the best-selling drug in the world.

An advert in the *Archives of General Psychiatry* in 1970[8] depicted Jan, 'single and psychoneurotic' because 'she had never found a man to match up to her father', as the ideal candidate for Valium.

Nevertheless, possible causes other than inherent 'psychoneuroses' occurred to me often, as I listened, in the 1980s, to the stories told by many women in the hospital where I trained as a psychiatrist. I wondered if their problems didn't lie *within* them but instead within their *relationships*, with their families, and especially the men in their lives.

My consultant boss prescribed more or different medication and even courses of ECT to improve their mood. It was a period when a *great deal* of electroconvulsive therapy was still administered (it's *still* used but much less now, see Chapter 12), and I remember having a daily list of 15 to 20 patients waiting in a large room in the hospital to have the treatment.

'She will be much happier again with her husband when she is *better*,' I remember being told when I raised the question of unhappy marriage as a possible cause. And some indeed were. But for others the relationship problems continued, and nothing changed. The women remained low in spirits *despite* the treatment.

By then the 'problem' was firmly called Depression.

And, as time moved on towards the 1990s, drug companies began to publicise their new wonder drug and to persuade doctors to identify more depression. It was promoted as safer than the older antidepressant drugs and set to become a global phenomenon: Prozac.

Now women are diagnosed with depression at almost twice the rate of men.[9]

Depression or Unhappiness?

In her book *The Madness of Women*, Professor Jane Ussher refers to depression as 'the daughter of hysteria'. She believes that 'reifying' unhappiness and distress as a 'pathological condition' serves to legitimise using psychiatric drugs to treat it.[10]

However, as medical historians have shown,[11] 'depression' is far from a new phenomenon, even if the marketing of drugs promoted its use as a diagnosis *very aggressively* in the last part of the twentieth century. There is no single 'thing' called 'major depression', and the experience of depression varies tremendously between individuals. But what they have in common is a profound, deep and lingering sense of sadness and sorrow, which can reach the point that they no longer feel that life is worth living. Sylvia Plath, who lived and died only a short way from Hannah Gavron in London, described an experience of life ceasing under the eponymous bell jar, while the world outside continued like a bad dream.[12] This conjures up an image of something much more than unhappiness.

Some people will say 'depressive illness' fits their experience, but these words just don't feel 'right' for others. And although biology plays a part, there isn't much biological evidence to explain the difference in rates of diagnosis beyond the influence of hormones on our mood.

So why do women get diagnosed with depression more often than men?

There are two possibilities. First, women are simply more likely to be *labelled* as depressed than men. Second, women are more *vulnerable* to depression than men.[13] Although they sound contradictory, both are probably true. Women *are* more likely to consult doctors asking for help more often than men, and when they ask for help with 'medically unexplained' physical symptoms, for which no physical cause is obvious, they may simply be dismissed with, 'there's nothing wrong with you, you are *just* depressed'. As a researcher in the 1980s, I would sometimes see the letters 'TATT CC AAO' in doctors' case records. I soon learned this was shorthand for 'tired all the time, can't cope, aching all over', and really didn't say much for the understanding of the medical profession for women's life problems.

But there is also evidence that women experience both more distress *and* depression, and this is strongly related to the kind of lives we lead.

What happens in women's early lives[14] such as abuse, family separation, death of parents, lack of support or single parenthood makes women more vulnerable. A family history also adds to the risk of getting depressed, as it did for me. Our early experiences may not only affect self-esteem and sense of being able to control our lives, but also the way our minds and bodies respond to stresses. Balance of *stress* and *support* is crucial. For example, we know that for women living in an urban setting, losing your mother early in life, having a partner you can't confide in, three small children under the age of 5 to care for, and no work outside the home, all increase the risk of you getting depressed.[15] What a surprise! Then experiencing life events and losses may trigger depression, and for vulnerable women in more traditional relationships, it's particularly events to do with children and families that matter.

Any of these events would make you feel miserable, wouldn't they? Of course, but not everyone gets depressed. Some of us do, but others are remarkably resilient, and it's the interplay between vulnerability and life events that is key here.

Poverty can make it so much harder to escape from difficult relationships and domestic violence. Working-class women get depressed more often than middle-class women, because they are *more likely* to experience the kind of life events that trigger depression.

But this alone was never sufficient to explain why *this* woman sitting in from of me in *this* clinic was seriously depressed *now*.

Emotional Work

Women still take much of the responsibility for the emotional work that has to be done in relationships and families, *especially* in the more traditional ones.

Disappointment in relationships was at the heart of the mental health problems of many women I saw in my career, along with trying and failing to cope with losses such as a miscarriage, bereavement, or repossession of a home. These, especially for more vulnerable women with a past or family history of depression, or a history of early trauma, could lead to depression.

I have met women still grieving quietly for the child they lost 30 years ago and unable to talk about it for fear of upsetting the family, and women pining for their son serving a long prison sentence whom they will never, ever give up on. Their partners, however, were more absorbed by their work, their mates and their hobbies.

My father had a shed-full of hobbies that absorbed him.

My mother had none. There was no 'after work'. She carried the emotional burden of keeping the family going, while my father tinkered with his tools, satisfied that he had already 'done a day's hard work', even though Mum went *out* to work too, spending all day behind the counter in a shop.

Men may be remarkably unaware that their wives and girlfriends want more.

As the feminist writer bell hooks put it so succinctly, 'most men feel they receive love and therefore know what it's like to be loved; women often feel we are in a constant state of yearning. Wanting love but not receiving it.'[16]

After escaping from a difficult and violent first marriage (see Chapter 6) in which she was chronically depressed, Amrah, who herself came from an abusive home, struggled with loneliness. Eventually she re-married a divorcee she met through a friend: 'I thought maybe I should give it a chance.'

They had 12 very good years together. They had a son. Then she learned he had also started to have a relationship with someone who she considered as a friend, and she felt utterly betrayed and bereft. She is still very, very angry: 'I trusted him too much.'

When we spoke, they were still together. She was still trying to forgive. He was expressing guilt, but she was feeling very depressed again, and having counselling once more.

When women get angry and respond emotionally, being 'emotional' is then seen as a handicap, instead of being *rational*, like men.

Out of their minds.

Liliana Pasterska is a Polish-born psychiatrist who spent many years working with women. We met up again when we both went to listen to Susie Orbach and Luise Eichenbaum talk about relationship problems. A day which marked 30 years after I first went along to that fateful weekend at the Women's Therapy Centre, and learned it wasn't easy to be accepted as both a psychiatrist and a feminist.

When we spoke later, Liliana said, 'There is a lot of emotional growing up we all have to do in relation to life, how it changes and what it throws at us. Maturing with our children affords one such opportunity – *no longer* the traditional privilege of women only.'

She was right. It *doesn't* always have to be women doing all the emotional work. And true partnerships do exist.

When Sally (in Chapter 4) experienced severe post-natal depression, her husband kept everything going valiantly, providing Sally with all the support she needed. Finally, he admitted he was struggling to cope too, and they went to see a therapist together.

She told me, 'We were talking about what had happened and my husband just burst into tears. And he was hyperventilating. And I'd *never seen* that.'

He hadn't felt supported throughout Sally's long hospital stay. The post-natal depression group started a father's group but only one other partner turned up. It fizzled out soon after.

They arrived at a decision together not to have more children, and Sally's husband had a vasectomy. They were able to be open and honest with each other.

But if it isn't a true partnership where painful emotions can be shared, and life problems such as loss of children, poor health and loss of trust in the relationship are talked through, women can feel very stuck, trapped and get depressed. It can happen the other way around too, but even today, our society is still remarkably paternalistic, with traditional division of roles. The psychoanalyst Carl Jung noted that 'where the will to power is paramount, love will be lacking'.[17] And if we have never experienced that kind of nurturing love early in life, it can be harder to both give and receive it later in our lives.

Reflecting on both her long and companionable marriage and her professional work, Liliana told me:

> Relationships make things possible . . . or impossible. If there is a rigid attitude to the division of roles, this can cause a problem.
>
> Women with whom I worked tended to have a powerful sense of responsibility not only for their families, but also for their jobs outside the home too. This could create a feeling of being trapped, should the systems at work, and/or at home, just not be flexible enough.

Paternalistic views have changed considerably in the last 50 years, but systemic changes are slower and less influenced by individual attitudes.

And women's emotional work extends way beyond the home and family into the workplace.

Keira, who is in her thirties now, learned early in life that there wasn't time to talk about feelings. In a family beset by early bereavement, chronic illness and addictions, she struggled with depression, anxiety, self-harm and suicidal thoughts through her teens and early twenties: 'My Mum was very much of the mindset, "You don't see me crying about it, my husband's dead, and I'm fine. What are you moping about?"'

When depression and anxiety start early, in adolescence, women are much more likely to go on to have episodes in adult life.

That was certainly true for Keira, but just as for many women I have known, it fuelled her desire to care for others:

> For a long time, I felt I needed to prevent anyone else from experiencing distress. It felt so overwhelming and horrific for me, that I couldn't bear the idea that anyone else was upset. So, I was one of those really irritating people that wants to swoop in and fix everything for everyone else.
>
> Women feel the need to nurture. They can get overly involved and become very overwhelmed by that.

But that didn't stop her, and after having therapy for herself, she began to train in it.

So many young people, especially women, still take psychology at university to 'try and understand themselves'. It doesn't work that way, but they go on to work in the caring professions, as I did. 'Women's work' was how my boss, a professor, described the therapy I was learning to offer my patients as a junior doctor. Not 'hard science' or 'serious medicine to do with drugs', but the act of listening and talking with people. The 'soft' skills we apparently excel at which are crucial to keeping everyone going. We are trained to care from an early age. Taking care of people's emotional lives really does matter, but it is undervalued, like all kinds of caring work.

And almost all the therapists in the audience, the day I met up with Liliana in London for a day about 'relationships', were women. Some of the leaders of change in the second wave of feminism trained as therapists themselves in the traditional schools of psychotherapy.[18] Meanwhile, the 'softer' attitudes and skills that women brought to the workplace were taken on by institutions and organisations. Women *are* better at building relationships, talking about emotions, and working in teams – important in a world that no longer depends so much on the brute physical strength needed for the manual labour that my parents' generation did.

However, they are still exploited.

Hard Labour

In *The Feminine Mystique*, Betty Frieden didn't discuss whether it was more fulfilling to do repetitive, exhausting work for low pay than to be a 'stay at home' housewife.

When Hannah Gavron interviewed women in Kentish Town, London, in the 1960s, middle-class women were beginning to work much more outside the home, having previously given up jobs after marriage. It wasn't just about income, it was about taking the opportunity to regain their independence and achieve their aspirations, which was very positive for them. However, this was nothing new for many women from the working classes, who had worked to supplement the family income for generations. For both, that meant 'juggling' being a housewife and mother as well as an employee.

How much has changed since then?

Even though housework today *is* shared much more than in the past, the average heterosexual British woman *still* puts in more than 12 days of household labour a year than her male companion.[19] And for many women 'work' still means hard labour, sometimes in multiple jobs simply to keep their families alive, yet also taking major responsibility for the household and family.

Women today in the workplace are still valued for our 'nimble little fingers' for stitching tee shirts, even ironically the ones that say 'This is what a Feminist looks like', at rock bottom wages in third (and first) world sweatshops. Not so very different from the skills my mother used to pod peas and 'top-and-tail' Brussels sprouts in the frozen vegetable factory when I was a child.

In *Nickel and Dimed*,[20] the journalist Barbara Ehrenreich chronicled her attempt to live on subsistence wages in America doing the jobs that women are so often barely noticed doing in our society, except when they are no longer there, such as cleaning houses and care work. She found herself working alongside women in chronic pain from arthritis and injuries but who could not afford to have time off. These are physically punishing jobs that damage your health if you have to do them year after year, two or more at a time just to survive.

And when it comes to the low-paid jobs that require 'people' skills, we are in constant demand, and under pressure to meet targets, which can harm our mental health.

Sally tried to return to her job in a call centre when she had recovered from post-natal depression but found it very difficult. Previously she had been able to handle calls where she could have proper conversations with customers but then there were cutbacks in the system.

'You were put in a seat, given a headset, and told to take calls. Now I remember thinking, I don't want to do this. There was a script. They had just stripped away everything else. You sat and looked at a screen that told you how many calls there were in the queue.'

There was a breakout space that she asked to use after a very difficult call. The screen said another 50 were waiting.

Her supervisor refused.

She couldn't go on. 'I just slipped off my headset and threw it down and went outside to walk. And I came back in and said to them, *I can't do this.*'

When Covid-19 struck, we discovered, if we didn't know already, that the jobs we had fought so hard for were still not valued as much as those of men, as it was women who mostly had to cope with the impact of Covid on the family.

A survey of women at work during the pandemic by LeanIn, an advocacy group for working women in the USA (taking its name from the ultimate corporate feminist book), found that nearly 1 in 3 women working full time with a partner and children felt that they had more to do than they could possibly handle, compared to about 1 in 8 men in the same situation[21] and the burden of caring for sick or elderly relatives was two or three times greater in hours per week for Black and Latinx women than white women.[22]

In health care, where 67% of employees worldwide are women, the gender pay gap is not only 24 percentage points in favour of men, but the impact of Covid-19 disproportionately affected lower paid workers, most of whom are women.[23]

When we spoke in May 2020, during the first lockdown in England, Susie Orbach said: 'What Covid has really opened up is showing how *much* labour women are doing all the time.' Not only what they usually did anyway between house and home but also home-schooling now.

'Feminists were absolutely determined to change the nature of *work*. I mean, we didn't succeed but we wanted to change it. We didn't want to be in little boxes doing corporate accounting.'

However, the successful women of my generation and afterwards weren't concerned with changing the nature of work but competing to get the best job they could and building a career. In 1984, bell hooks noted how so many liberal feminist reforms simply reinforced capitalist values without having any positive impact on women economically.[24]

As a young doctor, 40 years ago, I was competing with other women even though women held no positions of power in organisations. And whilst doing that we had to deal with everyday sexism in the workplace. I worked for a surgeon who refused to speak directly to me because he disapproved of women doctors. His instructions had, instead, to be relayed by the ward sister. It's so depressing to find that even now, on social media, many women doctors report having similar experiences.

My friend Samantha, now in her forties and working in West Coast corporate America, says she *still* has to deal with 'unreconstructed men' at work. This leaves her so angry.

'I don't want to be helped by men. I just want them to stop being assholes. It's their problem.'

Then, when the pandemic arrived we all found out that our failure to change what society understood by 'work' meant that all of the sustaining, caring and nurturing carried out largely by women and still unrecognised and rewarded by society (and completely invisible to corporate feminism) actually still remained 'our responsibility'. It must have come as a shock to many women who had steadfastly been building their careers.

As Kim Brooks questioned in a *New York Times* opinion piece,[25] if the pandemic undid our three decades of progress on gender equality, then how real was that progress?

For *many* women across the world? Not very real at all.

Trying to Cope

We all have ways of coping with pressure, stresses and life events and work. Women *are* better at seeking support and talking things over with others than men, but we also have a history of using other, less healthy and acceptable means of coping: sedatives and alcohol. Just think of the derogatory terms for them: 'Mother's little helpers' for, diazepam (Valium) and 'Mother's ruin', for gin.

Rachel Bannister, who told me about the prolonged struggle to find help for her daughter's anorexia (see Chapter 3), has written about the serious addiction she developed to the benzodiazepine, temazepam (similar to Valium) in liquid form, during that period.

'For me, the liquid temazepam was a desperate and ultimately destructive means to alleviate great internal pain and trauma. Pain relief for what I describe as feeling like a "hole in my soul".'[26]

She told me later, 'I had this GP who just kept giving it me, and he did actually get struck off in the end. He said "You'll be alright you've got three beautiful girls. See you when you want your prescription again!"'

Dee, in her twenties and newly working in public relations, had never drunk alcohol until she found herself in a job where she had to sometimes deal with difficult people in business meetings, and alcohol was freely available.

'It's amazing how alcohol slips from being something that's very helpful in your life, to something that you can't control.'

I've used it myself far too much in the past to help with my anxiety, and I've treated many women for depression who started drinking alcohol only to be able to sleep. But women who drink heavily are judged differently from men.

'If a woman gets drunk, she's just cheap, you know?'

Like Dee, I remember drinking heavily in my youth to prove I could equal the men. But then, as Dee put it, they'd probably be thinking, but not saying, 'You're a woman and we quite like women really being *women.*'

Well behaved.

Clinical psychologist Annie Hickox, who has written about depression in her own family, says, 'Both men and women ask for help because they want to be functioning as well as they can.' But women seek help from doctors because they are not only struggling personally but are also painfully aware of the negative impact of that on their families and those around them.[27]

'I see a lot more anxieties about their health in women than in men, and I think that's to do with feeling very vulnerable.'

My friend Professor Carolyn Chew-Graham has been a GP in Manchester for more than 30 years. She said there isn't really a big gender difference in how younger people talk to her about depression and anxiety, but older women *are* more open to discussing it than men.

And doctors vary enormously.

'Some may miss depression and others diagnose it when it's not there.'

She firmly believes a diagnosis *must* be negotiated with the patient but acknowledges it isn't always.

'I'll say . . . "I wonder whether you're depressed, what do you think about that?"'

Women then follow-through with seeking therapy much more than men do.

'But most people seem to just get CBT. Whether they want it or not, or whether I think it would be useful at all.' The alternatives – *different* kinds of therapy – can be difficult to access unless you pay, with waits of more than a year on the NHS.

I could sense Carolyn's deep frustration at a system that fails to provide what it should be able to. It's extraordinarily difficult in the UK to access the kind of longer- term psychotherapeutic help that you need to deal with the impact of early life events and relationships unless you pay. And easy to end up having your persistent depression relabelled as 'personality disorder'.

Antidepressants *and* therapy together are recommended for more severe depression.[28] Twice as many women as men get prescribed antidepressants,[29] simply because we are twice as likely to get diagnosed with depression, and even though pharmaceutical companies massively promoted these pills to doctors in the past, they *do* work for many. I don't think I'd still be here without them, and I certainly wouldn't have been able to engage with all the psychotherapy I had too. There were times I couldn't get out of bed or read a book. But some are not helped at all.

'I felt 1000 times worse in terms of like suicidal ideas and not wanting to be here and struggling,' Keira, who later trained as a therapist herself, told me. 'I was really violently sick. My legs were like jelly constantly.'

In contrast, Sally took them with considerable benefit and recovered from post-natal depression but said, 'Psychiatrists and GPs don't take account of the problem that gaining weight is for women.'

I should add in here that there *are* other problems too with taking antidepressants for depression. Doctors don't say much about the lack of sexual desire that antidepressants can cause,[30] perhaps because it can be hard to distinguish what's caused by the tablets and what's a residual effect of the depression. There is also continual concern about the risk of addiction. Antidepressants can be difficult to withdraw from, and it *must* be done slowly. It's too easy to get left on them for years.

But what else, apart from pills, and brief therapy, is there to offer women help with the life problems that increase their risk of depression? Those endless cycles of exhausting emotional and physical work. *Very little* that is designed around what *women* need. Support, a place to help each other, to reflect on how to change their lives for the better. There is specific help for domestic violence, yes, but many women's centres and organisations such as the Women's Therapy Centre I visited in the 1980s in North London closed during the period of austerity after the economic crash of 2008.[31]

'Help' focuses on getting you feeling better, but not much on assisting you to make changes to your life so that you can really recover and remain well.

That takes longer than four to six sessions.

What Must Change?

Where do I begin?

When I asked Carolyn, my GP friend, that question, she replied, 'It's about women's roles being valued in society. Not objectified.'

And she is right. These are core problems for women that we've been fighting for so long. We are told that we should value ourselves, that we don't have enough self-esteem. The problem lies inside us not society. We fall into what Jessa Crispin in *Why I Am Not A Feminist*[32] calls the 'trap of the self-help mindset' and spend time working on our 'faults'.

So focused are we on our 'selves' that what we don't seem to do enough of is to value *each other* as women. Not only providing mutual support and sharing our stories but also fighting to improve the lot of those women who have made it possible for some of us to have careers and exciting lives by cleaning our floors and taking care of our children. Once we met up regularly in 'consciousness raising groups' in each other's homes, to share support, encouragement and knowledge. They are no more.

But many of us *do* now meet up online. Many of the women I have met in the last decade on social media have not only supported me but also contributed to this book.

In the second wave of feminism, women founded organisations *for women*. Self-Injury Support in Bristol was one of those, founded by a group of women in 1988 who wanted to do something positive for women who self-injure in their community, and it is still going strong! When a friend, a psychiatrist from Brazil, came to visit me in Manchester, she asked where all the grassroots organisations founded by women for women were in the area I worked, and was surprised we had so few.

In many ways it would be harder now than it was in 1988 to start up such an enterprise as the issue of gender has so divided feminism and seems to have almost paralysed our ability to move forwards.

But we must find a way.

If *we* don't do it, we can't expect men to lead on it, ever.

Our health care systems largely ignore the massive part that gender plays in why more women than men get depressed. This is not denying that men have problems, of course they do, but in the UK all the focus is currently on male suicide and getting men to talk. Women need to talk too about the reasons why they are suffering, but there are fewer places than ever where they can get the kind of help that they need to make changes in their lives, where there is therapy that lasts long enough to make a difference.

As women today, we must take the lead in creating and running such places, as our mothers and grandmothers did.

It sometimes feels like feminism is unable to move on from the past crimes of psychiatry against women and that's understandable *to a point*. But we need to find better ways of helping women who are suffering *now*, which don't only focus on their victimhood and oppression. Whatever some would like to believe, that includes antidepressants for those who do benefit from them.

Annie Hickox is not only a a clinical psychologist but also a feminist, and has strong views on this: 'Denying women's vulnerability to mental illness, denying the diagnosis of "depression", overzealously categorising everything we suffer as trauma or due to the patriarchy is not a way to end sexism and it's not empowering.'

As a psychiatrist, what *I have* learned from feminism is that understanding women's mental health and illness in the round, looking through the three lenses of biological, psychological and social factors that all play a part is simply not enough.[33] We *must* also look through the *fourth* lens that focuses on the powerful economic and political forces that impact negatively on women's lives to fully understand why women experience an excess of anxiety and depression[34] in our societies and to make real changes.

That means getting health professionals to step outside the door of the clinic into the wider world and engage with what is happening there: supporting grassroots organisations, listening to them and getting their voices heard in the community.

Professionals often don't believe they possess much power.

But really, they do.

We must encourage them to use it.

Hannah Gavron's book, which was published in 1965, was one of the first feminist explorations of the conflicts that women face between work outside the home, and their roles and work within it as wives and mothers.

Despite its complete failure to address the lives of women beyond the white, middle and upper classes, Betty Friedan's writing did help to trigger a revolution that changed the world for many. Including me.

But, for women like Hannah, it was already too late.

6

·····

Unheard, Ignored, Entrapped?

'I don't know anyone to whom I would have to explain about being followed around in shops, because it happens all the time, to me and every other Black person that I know.'

Professor Dawn Edge is the University of Manchester's first Black, female professor. When she told me about her lifelong daily experience of racism, I was both shocked and saddened that it had *never occurred to me* this might happen to her.

'If that is the case,' I asked myself, 'How can I even attempt to write about the experience of Black and ethnic minoritised women?'

'Should I even be trying to?'

I'm sure there are some who'd immediately say 'no'.

I remember someone in the audience at the debate that evening in Manchester shouting out, 'Would all of the speakers please care to check their privilege?'

At the time I was offended. I'm a white, working-class woman who managed to claw her way up to be a professor too, at the medical school in Manchester, when that was so unusual for a woman that people would come to interview me (and others like me) to try to understand how that was even possible.

I replied, 'I'm fortunate, not privileged.'

Looking around I made eye contact with the person in the audience who had said it. She gave me a knowing smile.

I consider my privilege differently now. Despite coming from the working classes, I can acknowledge I've always had *white* privilege. Life would have been even harder if I'd been Black. I'm very middle class these days and in possession of the power to do and say things that many other women still cannot.

I'm also a psychiatrist of a kind, I hope, that seeks to understand how and why a person comes to think and feel the way that she does about herself, the world and the future, rather than pass judgement.

In 1984, it was the Black feminist writer bell hooks who said of Betty Friedan that she had written as though women of other races and classes, those *most* victimised by sexist oppression, simply didn't exist.[1] And it was the Black feminist law professor Kimberlé Crenshaw who coined the term 'intersectionality'.[2] The *intersecting* categories of discrimination and oppression – gender, race, class, sexual orientation and physical ability – that contribute to women's differing degrees of privilege.

Not long after the millennium, an older woman, who I knew was a holocaust survivor, asked me in the clinic, 'Are you Jewish? If you aren't, I don't think you can understand what I've been through.'

'No', I'm not,' I replied. 'But I'm here to listen, to learn and to work out how I can help. Is that OK with you?'

Since then, I've learned a great deal.

About how white feminists failed their Black sisters repeatedly in the last century, arguing that white women deserved the vote before Black men, and later refusing to accept their own complicity in racism and the oppression of Black women.[3] How 'Black feminism' was largely excluded from the history of the 'waves' of feminism written by white, middle-class academics.

Women like me.[4]

I've been listening to, and learning from, women who feel both unheard and discriminated against, and what they have told me about is racism.

Living with Racism

In North Carolina, during the 1940s, Eunice Waymon had a dream. Something she had been working towards all her young life. It was to become the first great Black American classical pianist.

Only one day in August 1950, in Philadelphia, that dream ended. After years of preparation, she was rejected at her audition for the Curtis Institute of Music. We will never know whether it was because she was Black and female. The institute of course denied this. But Eunice herself believed it was because she was a poor, unknown, Black girl and the rejection had a lifelong impact on her.[5]

Eunice Waymon would later become Nina Simone, one of the most talented musical performers of the twentieth century.

Racism is the system by which the dominant *white* group in our society categorises individuals into races then devalues and disempowers them.[6]

Living with racism affects women's lives in so many different ways, from the rejection that Nina Simone experienced to the impact of racist judgements about what is considered 'beautiful' in society, to simply getting access to education. Then there is being repeatedly subject to explicit racism in everyday life. It's different for women of different colours: Black, Asian, Latino. Gender and race then intersect with socioeconomic class.

But there is a hierarchy, and poor Black women are at the bottom of it.

Freida, who grew up in financial hardship in Chicago in the 1960s, told me she had no doubt that racism played a part in her mental health problems. She's had treatment for panic attacks and depression over many years.

'Black people do struggle. I think that's been part of the reason why they suffer with depression. Because of the way they are treated. Because of the colour of their skin. I'm so dark skinned I got teased a lot when I was a child. Called Black Sambo, Black Spook. I thought of myself as ugly.'

Listening to Freida I recalled that in the book *Living While Black*, Guilaine Kinounani, a Black, French psychologist, describes how a cousin bought her child a Black doll as a gift, only for her to reject it as 'ugly'.[7] The little girl had already learned at a very young age that white was prettier. In the same way, Freida both judged herself, by internalising that racism, and was judged by school bullies as being well down the scale of attractiveness because of her darker skin. She was considered to be of less intrinsic worth and, as a result, of attractiveness. Freida was right: racism seriously affected her self-esteem early in life and increased her vulnerability to depression later.

My colleague Bushra Nazir, who has researched mental health problems in South Asian women, told me about her own experiences at school as a British South Asian, growing up in Manchester in the 1990s. Asian girls were discriminated against by staff, who assumed they didn't need to learn anything.

'One of the teachers said to a group of us, "Oh, you're just going to get married, aren't you? There's no point me teaching you. I think you should sit right at the back of the class", which we did. And I think my education did suffer. I didn't get the attention.'

Bushra and her friends were fitted to a stereotype of an Asian girl who would be merely sent away from home and married off young.

Someone of little value.

In contrast, Sylvia, who is half-Filipino, grew up in a very white, insular, upper middle-class suburb on the East Coast of America in the early twenty-first century. Sheltered by the wealth of her family, she was unaware of any racial tensions during her childhood.

'There was a lot of background academic pressure. My parents were very aware of it and didn't want to be categorised as "Tiger" parents (a stereotype for ambitious Asian mothers in particular). But the expectations were still there.'

She began to suffer with panic attacks at the age of 13 after the death of a close family friend and Sylvia's parents paid for her to get therapy. However, they didn't think it was any more than school-related stress, despite a family history of more severe depression:

> I don't think I realised that the adults I grew up around were so conservative until Trump was elected. That's when things started coming out. There were people who said they didn't consider my mom a person of colour because she was a *friend*. It was just very strange to have that realisation about the context I was raised in.
>
> My brother gets more explicit racism, but I doubt he gets as many questions as *Where are you from?* How long have you been in America. I've gotten that my entire life.

And for Sylvia, that daily harassment on the street, so frequent for young women, comes with added racist overtones too.

For each of these women, being a *woman of colour* has added an additional dimension of difficulties to their experience of living in the world, but Freida's story has a further twist. Now in her sixties, not only has she experienced racism during her working life, but she also found it impossible to report the two occasions she had been sexually assaulted to the police.

'I didn't. Because I'm a woman who was Black. And I had a child out of wedlock. And I figured if one guy had a really good job working for electronics company, and other guy was a fireman, I'm thinking the police were going to believe them before they believed me.'

Freida was poor, an unmarried mother, which was also highly stigmatised in her community at that time, and Black. She did not think she would be heard or believed.

She didn't tell anyone at all for many years.

But the impact of racism *and* sexism is more than simply additive. Women of colour experience *gendered racism*. Prejudice, harassment and violence and distinctive sexist stereotyping by race: Black women are 'unfeminine, aggressive and strong' (and in the USA they are also seen as 'sassy' and sexual so perhaps even 'asking' for assault); Asian women are 'passive and sexually exotic'; Latina women are stereotyped as 'maids' and 'housekeepers'; while white women are seen as both 'passive' and 'confident', in keeping, of course, with both male and white supremacy. Rigid stereotypes shape not only what happens to women of colour but also the barriers they face in seeking help.[8]

Freida didn't speak about the assaults for many years. She feared not being heard. They have had a lifelong impact on her mental health.

Racism Harms Mental Health

Lade Smith is now president of the Royal College of Psychiatrists in the UK. She told me what happened to her only a couple of days before we met on Zoom:

> I was at a conference. It was lunchtime. There were people dressed in white shirts and black trousers, and *obviously* waiters, doing the clearing up. I was wearing a blue dress and a big green coat, and I went to sit down near a table, and a delegate standing nearby said to me, 'Oh, it's okay. You can take those plates away now.'
>
> I just looked at him to see if he realised that I was so obviously not a waiter, but he didn't because *all he could see was the blackface*. And then having seen that I didn't move the plates, he just harrumphed and did it himself. But he couldn't even acknowledge the mistake he'd made, because he didn't think that the kind of person that *he thought I was* in his head was someone even worthy of that common apology. That was, in some ways, even more of an insult.
>
> And it happens all the time.

We've already talked about things such as genetics, early life experiences and poverty. These things make us vulnerable to mental illness. Add to that the constant reminder that you are not as *valued* as other people:

> Every insult is a small, emotional trauma that happens regularly. It can take its toll on people. And depending on your temperament, or whether you've got any of those biological factors that are important and on your familial environment – if you've been supported and loved, or emotionally neglected – they may or may not contribute to you becoming unwell.

There's probably only so much that people can take.

Nina Simone would have experienced many such racist slurs throughout her life.

In his book *What Happened Miss Simone?*, Alan Light describes how, in her first recital, Nina's parents were moved away from the front row to make way for white audience members. Then there were the comments about her appearance. That her skin was too dark. Her lips too full. Her nose too big.

Much, much later she was diagnosed with bipolar disorder. How much of that was related to the repeated racism she experienced, her genetic inheritance, or the quite stark lack of love and support from her mother, a religious woman who disapproved of her daughter performing in nightclubs? Or her use of LSD?

They probably all played a part.

But for Black American women like Nina and Freida there *is* a clear association between race and experiencing anxiety, depression and post-traumatic stress disorder (PTSD).[9] Black women are 34% more likely to experience PTSD when compared with their white female counterparts.[10] Depression is not only more common, but it persists longer in women of Pakistani origin in the UK than either the white British population of either gender or men of Pakistani origin.[11] Black women in the UK are *more* likely to experience common mental health problems than white women[12] and *less* likely to be receiving treatment; however, Black people overall are four times more likely to be detained under the Mental Health Act.[13]

And there is a significant link between poorer physical and mental health and the kind of regular *racist* and *gendered* comments that Sylvia described,[14] sometimes called 'microaggressions'.

'I prefer plain English,' Lade said. 'I tell people how everyday insults can be traumatic and erode your sense of well-being.'

'It's such a *fundamental human need* to know that you in some way matter.

'However, Black men are feared, reviled and hated.

'And Black women are ignored.'

Invisible

When Dawn Edge wanted to talk to Black women for her PhD research on post-natal depression[15] in Manchester, she faced an immediate problem.

'I didn't know any Black women who talked about post-natal depression. And when I approached services, all of them said, *and they used the phrase,* "we don't see Black women". So, I was curious.'

Dawn eventually located pregnant Black women, who were feeling distressed and down in their mood, by visiting ante-natal services herself and engaging women via community groups and faith-based organisations.

Black and minoritised ethnic women are under-researched in comparison to men.

In addition to racism, they face greater social and economic inequalities such as homelessness and unemployment.[16] They are *more* likely to be lone parents[17] and are four times more likely to die in pregnancy and childbirth than white women, while Asian women are twice as likely.

Young, female, Black and minoritised ethnic doctors working in British mental health care are also more likely to experience racism too.[18]

All of this has consequences, for women, their children, and families.

But for some in our services, it is invisible.
We don't see Black women.

Elena, who is of both Afro-Caribbean and white descent, lost her mother suddenly to lung cancer at the age of 23. The grieving process was tough. She didn't know if what she was experiencing was normal, or not:

> There's also a lot of stigma around Black women being seen as quite strong and resilient. There's an expectation of not being vulnerable, not showing your weaknesses.
>
> You just do what you need to, deal with what is thrown at you and *be resilient*. Adapt to it. If you cry, or if you're sad, it's a sign of weakness. That is something that is still in me now. I'm struggling to unlearn it.

The first port of call for many Black, Asian, and other minoritised ethnic women may be the church, the temple, synagogue or the Imam. Or people may simply say, 'that's just how they are', when someone is behaving differently or distressed.

But, as Lade Smith said, 'The problem is that when people *do* feel that it's illness, they don't always feel safe going to mental health services.'

This is hardly surprising given the negative experiences that Black and minority communities have had with mental health care over decades. There is real terror of being forever trapped and 'lost within the system'.

Dawn Edge said the pregnant women she spoke to were *fearful* of being diagnosed with depression: 'They wouldn't use the D-word, they might start off with a "d. . ." and then talk about feeling down or feeling flat. *Any* other word to describe depressive feelings.'

This powerful taboo against 'depression' is reinforced if professionals say your problems are 'entirely understandable' given your circumstances, and say you *aren't distressed enough* for help from services. Not surprisingly, women will say, 'I knew that.'

'Putting it all down to the life you lead and brushing you off' is an attitude I recognise too, from the experiences of poor, white, working-class women with mental health services in the inner city. It's not just about race and gender, *class* plays a significant part too. Second-wave feminism had both a race and a class problem, and working-class women of colour are still at the bottom of the pile.

'If you've seen your GP or your midwife and they've told you that you're not depressed, and your life is just a bit shit, and you can't change anything what do you do then?

'You've just got to be strong, haven't you?'

Oppressed and Entrapped?

The sentiment that it is *culture* that is oppressive, not religion, is very familiar to me, particularly from many conversations with Islamic colleagues who have read the Qur'an for themselves and know what it does and does not say about women.

Yet, as someone who learned years ago, in an awkward moment of public rejection, that an orthodox Jewish doctor would not shake hands with me, a woman, in case I was currently menstruating, I wanted to know *more* about the specific role played by religion in oppression of women.

Francesca Stavrakopoulou, professor of Hebrew Bible and ancient religion at the University of Exeter, reiterated how important it was that we don't assume Western values are in any way superior.

'But,' she explained, 'it's beyond coincidence that in most traditional religious communities, including the Abrahamic faiths, that the power imbalance lies in favour of men.'

In other words, not just Islam but Judaism and Christianity too.

'And it's hugely damaging to women because they are automatically 'othered' in terms of their bodies. And the opposite is that men are valued.'

For many women, the impact of religion and culture is powerfully intertwined.

'We're different.

'We're treated differently by our own because we're women. We're treated differently outside because we're Asian.'

The words spoken by a 17-year-old South Asian girl to researchers in the north of England,[19] capturing the intersection between sexism *within* her home and racism *outside* of it.

Suicide rates in South Asian women in the UK are two and a half times those for white women, and those in the 16–24 age group, feeling trapped between two cultures, are particularly at risk. The burden of the family's honour or 'Izzat' is borne heavily by the women and reinforced by other women too: mothers, sisters, grandmothers. As 'cultural reproducers', women are used to ensure the longevity of patriarchy.[20]

Feelings of being under terrible pressure, isolated and unsupported lead to self-harming as a way of trying to cope, and even to suicide.

Twenty years ago, with a group of British Pakistani colleagues, mostly women, I was involved in trying to understand why British Pakistani women fail to recover from depression.[21] Listening to women living in the communities of terraced houses nestled around mosques in the mill towns of Lancashire, we heard not only about the impact of casual racism, sexual harassment at work and cross-cultural pressures, but also the strain caused by family rifts from which escape seemed impossible, such as arranged marriages between cousins which had subsequently broken down causing endless recriminations. My colleagues, well-educated Pakistani-born women who listened to painful stories told in a mixture of English, Punjabi and Urdu, were visibly shaken by what they heard and told me how life for South Asian women in working-class Lancashire often seemed more restrictive than in the wealthier cosmopolitan families they had grown up in abroad. Some had arranged marriages in which they were happy and content but were facing similar cross-cultural dilemmas with British-born daughters who were not prepared to meet family expectations.

Forced marriage, however, is something quite different altogether.

When Amrah was 17, she was taken with her 15-year-old sister to rural Bangladesh by her parents and told that she would be staying for several months and marrying her father's nephew. Any remaining teenage romantic expectations she had of love and companionship were rapidly extinguished.

'I told my parents I'd rather commit suicide than marry this guy. I'd try to hang myself, but they said, "Oh, she's not going to do it, she'll be OK."'

Her mother tried to persuade her: 'You'll have power. You have the passport. He'll treat you nice because he's ugly.'

Khatidja Chantler, who has researched forced marriage, told me women are often involved in doing the persuading: 'Not using physical force necessarily, but you could read it as coercive control, trying to persuade their daughters that a marriage is the only way.'

'After a while,' Amrah continued, 'I kind of accepted the situation. They wore me down. I said to them, "let me just get it done".'

Hoping to flee from a family where her father had been violent and controlling, she didn't expect things could be worse.

They were.

'I used to take my glasses off, so I didn't have to physically look at him. All I cared about was what colour paint I was going to put on the walls.'

Struggling with depression and anxiety she devoted her life instead to the three daughters that were a deep disappointment to both husband and father, who only wanted sons.

'He left the hospital when the last daughter was born. I was dumped because I was giving birth to a girl.'

It was several years before she was able to get a divorce.

In 2006 there were estimated to be around 5,000–8,000 forced marriages in England,[22] and that doesn't include the 'hidden' ones, the victims who do not come forward. Some 97% occurred in the Asian community, 96% of the victims were women and 41% were, like Amrah, under the age of 18.

Girls still disappear from school to be taken away and married.

Female genital mutilation (FGM), in which female external genitalia are either all or only partly removed, is another violation of the rights of women that the World Health Organisation estimates is done to 3 million girls every year in Africa alone.[23] No religion promotes or condones FGM. Yet, more than half of girls and women in four out of

14 countries where data are available saw FGM as a *religious* requirement, even though some religious leaders have spoken out against it.[24] It is illegal to carry it out in the UK, and there are now laws preventing girls being taken abroad to have it performed. The physical sequelae are bad enough: haemorrhage, infections, pain during sex and obstetric complications. We still know very little about the psychological impact, but it's likely to be similar in many ways to what other women subjected to patriarchal violence suffer (see Chapter 8).

Where religious faith has considerable power, women *are* subject to oppression, *simply for being women*, from Afghanistan to the Evangelical Southern states of the USA, and it plays a part in why women flee from both their families and their countries.

Rebecca Farrington, a GP in Manchester who has worked in refugee mental health care for several years, told me (with her permission) Sara's story.

'Sara is Iraqi Kurdish. And she's now 27. Her parents had a mixed marriage and she got married at 15, to a Kurdish man to cement her Kurdish identity, because she was getting bullied about her dad. And she had three children before she was 20.'

Sara's family escaped Iraq but her four-year-old daughter was shot and killed by a sniper.

'And she arrived utterly *devastated* by the idea that she was unable to keep her child safe.' She has never been able to engage with therapy for her PTSD; first because she was just too emotionally churned up, and then because it was so difficult to get through an inflexible system where she kept losing her place on the waiting list.

'First, she didn't understand the "opt-in" letter.' You must contact the clinic to say you want to attend the appointment. And you also must be here for 3 years before anyone will offer you a free English class.

Then she was given a time to attend when she also had to be at the children's school.

Two years passed. Sara became pregnant again.

'She was absolutely terrified of giving birth because *she didn't feel that she was able to keep her child safe.*'

Rebecca supported her through her pregnancy with several different midwives, a lack of interpreters, and an obstetrician who needed convincing to perform a caesarean section.

'And she's got an amazing relationship with this new baby.'

'But *now* her husband has decided that he wanted to go back to Iraq.' He is frustrated at not being able to work as their asylum claims have been unsuccessful.

'So, Sara told her health visitor that she was terrified, because in her culture, the man takes the children.

They're his.

'And she's *terrified* of going back.'

As a white British Feminist health professional, like Rebecca, I've struggled with views of those, such as Lola Olefemi,[25] Black feminist and author of *Feminism Interrupted*, who criticise the views and actions of 'white saviours', when I've been faced with situations in which women from an ethnic or religious minority, like Amrah and Sarah, are visibly suffering. I also *cannot* accept the view expressed by the prominent white feminist Germaine Greer that challenging FGM is an *attack on culture.*[26]

Khatidja Chantler's views on cultural relativism (the theory that beliefs, customs, and morality exist in relation to the culture from which they originate and are not absolute) were quite clear:

Professionals often see any type of abuse that's happening to Black and minoritised women through a cultural lens.

Well, just stop and think about that. If you're not going to intervene, because it's a cultural thing, it means you condone violence and abuse. How do you live with that? What's more important? Ensuring that a woman or a child can escape abuse? Or somebody's labelling me as being culturally insensitive?

Why am I even doing this job?

I challenge these *acts of violence* women are *suffering,* in *solidarity* with those women who are fighting this from *within* their own culture.

Women like Dr Hannana Siddiqui, who, with Southall Black Sisters, has fought for years to help women who are abused, forced to take their own lives, and murdered for the sake of 'honour'. She was vehement in her opinions:

> We've always been very critical of cultural relativism, and sensitivities around multicultural thinking – that you can't intervene in minority cultures or religions.
>
> We're not asking for cultural stereotypes. We're talking about a better understanding. It doesn't mean you're being racist when you intervene, it just means that you're protecting women who are vulnerable to abuse.
>
> They have rights as well.

Women have *universal human rights.*

Hannana told me how professionals have more courage to go forwards, in situations where they may fear criticism, when they have the support of an organisation like Southall Black Sisters, but that there are people within the community who don't like that, especially among the leaders who tend to be male and conservative.

But this is not to deny that Islamophobia is rife. It plays a considerable part in how Muslim women are both stereotypically painted as passive 'victims' and active 'terrorists' by society.

In *Inner Lives of Troubled Young Muslims,*[27] the journalist Yasmin Alibhai-Brown questions how, and why, young Muslim women like the four girls from Bethnal Green who travelled to Syria would want to leave their lives in London to join the caliphate? What made them so vulnerable to grooming? She finds potential answers in the conflicted and sometimes painful lives they were running from. Problems for which they were not only receiving no help, but which were unrecognised by those around them.

Hearing these young women's complex multi-layered life stories is key to understanding them.

Passing through Rebecca's clinic have been women fleeing from soldiers, domestic violence and persecution because of their sexuality. Women pregnant because of rape used as a form of torture. Professional women who have stood up against politicians for what they believed, and then suffered the consequences.

Some women prefer to be treated by women because of their religion. Some *only* want to see women because of what they have been through. Some are overwhelmed with shame and guilt for having left children behind them, and older family members whom they would have been expected to care for.

'Some feel incredibly regretful, although they know that staying wasn't an option either.

They struggle to feel safe too in the places they must live when they arrive here: hotels, shared houses. But they are *totally disempowered* by the system.'

In her clinic, Rebecca writes in letter after letter: 'I confirm this person has a diagnosis of post-traumatic stress disorder; these are the predominant symptoms. This is their treatment, and, in my opinion, *timely* resolution to their immigration claim will help their recovery.'

She has yet to find the magic words that will convey their need for certainty about their future safety.

An outcome without which healing will be very hard.

Healing

Healing is, in simple terms, the process of becoming healthy again. But it can mean many different things – not only restoration to physical health but also recovery in an emotional and spiritual way, by restoring energy, finding hope and a sense of meaning again in life. It can also take place on many different levels, from the individual overcoming their own doubts, uncertainties and problems either alone or within a therapeutic relationship, to healing which takes place within families, communities and cultures.

And how can professionals help?

When Black feminists began to organise in the UK in the 1960s, they rejected a feminism that was only about self and personal liberation but instead focused on rebuilding their communities. They targeted the appalling social and working conditions that were oppressing them. The famous strike at the Grunwick photo-processing plant, in 1976, was led by an extraordinarily determined South Asian woman, Jayaben Desai.[28] Audre Lorde spoke in *Sister Outsider* of how there is no such thing as a single-issue fight, because none of us lead single-issue lives.[29]

At first, little of this grassroots wisdom filtered through to the lives that I and other white British feminists led in the 1980s in our middle-class women's groups. But for me, the voice of Maya Angelou reading her poem 'And still I rise' was a beacon in the darkness when I had all but lost hope after a broken relationship. It helped me to heal.

Black women's mental health and wellbeing is an important focus for Black feminism. Audre Lorde emphasised the importance of poetry[30] to engage with feelings, dreams and fears. Other Black feminist writers such as bell hooks, Kimberlé Crenshaw, Ntgoze Shange, Toni Morrison and Alice Walker all contributed to a body of work that affirms Black womanhood – her strength, power and unique position – that for me is embodied in Maya Angelou's marvellous poem 'Phenomenal Woman'.

How does the concept of 'mental illness', and the sometimes controversial practices of psychiatric diagnosis and treatment, fit with this view of personal healing that focuses on emotional and spiritual growth and overcoming oppression rather than diagnosis and treatment?

Chimamanda Ngozi Adichie is an award-winning Nigerian author, famous for her Ted Talk 'We should all be feminists'.[31] She has also spoken about how she fell into a deep depression after writing her book *Half of the Yellow Sun*, based on her own family's experiences in the Biafran war.

When a powerful essay she had written on depression was published in 2015 in *The Guardian*, but quickly withdrawn because she said she had *not* intended for it to be published at that point, her management released a statement which said: 'Depression is a very important subject for her ... many people suffer in silence. Breaking the silence around the subject of depression can be the first step to getting better.' [32]

Reading this, I remembered how in our conversation, Professor Dawn Edge cautioned that, 'If a Black woman tells a health care professional that she's depressed, she *has* tried everything else.'

However, the psychologist Guilliane Kinouani, commenting on Adichie's article, asked in a subsequent blog[33] whether depression *is* a useful word for Black women, and expressed her hope that Adichie might also give credence to other more afrocentric models of mental health.

Kinouani's 2021 book *Living While Black* is based on her considerable clinical experience of helping people to overcome racial trauma. It's an extraordinary read, drawing from history, culture and science, and encourages the reader to begin their own self-care. Along with other psychiatric diagnoses, depression remains contested, and may be seen as the *language of oppression* – of a colonial, Western psychiatry and psychology, which have undoubtedly been both institutionally racist and sexist.[34] Diagnosis, and in particular the diagnosis of depression, can be a helpful concept for some women, whatever their culture, but not for everyone.

Sylvia told me that after receiving many different diagnoses over the years she finds her diagnosis of bipolar 2 disorder helpful to a point.

'But I think diagnoses are very limiting. The important thing is that it remains on my chart, so nobody takes me off my mood stabiliser ever. Because that's the one thing that *has* definitely helped!'

Diagnosis can be helpful as it indicates what treatment is likely to help. But *no one* should have to accept a diagnostic label to receive care. 'Depression' is *not* an acceptable word for many people, and we should be exploring and negotiating the words and ideas that feel right for *this* person, *here and now* in conversation with them. I worked with women who found the idea of depression and other Western diagnoses completely unacceptable and wanted to find their own non-medical ways of healing. Sometimes both Western medicine and Eastern spiritual remedies were combined. Sometimes we agreed to hold my medicines and therapies in reserve to use if there was no improvement. I tried to listen and most of all respect that people may have different beliefs and experiences, but I know I did not always succeed.

And, though I may have felt that I could *attempt* to understand the experiences of the Jewish holocaust survivor in the clinic, I now acknowledge my essential naivety.

As Rebecca Farrington told me, '*Cultural humility* is vital.'

And cultural knowledge is several generations deep.

I've personally helped to set up services that reach out to women in the South Asian and the Jewish communities in Manchester, and I've learned how, for most, having psychological therapy with someone from the same culture is important too. But not always possible. I've also met women who would prefer to talk to a white British therapist through an interpreter because of their fears about confidentiality, or because they want to talk about something which may be culturally problematic, like sexuality and gender. But services and therapists that succeed in reaching out to Black and minoritised ethnic women use language, stories and ideas that are familiar and 'fit' with their own experience of their lives.

The sharing of stories and experiences between Black women is crucial to Suryia Nayak's work both at the grassroots and in academia. Originally trained as a social worker, the Manchester-based psychotherapist, academic and feminist has spent decades training in psychoanalysis, often as she puts it, as the 'odd one out' in a room mostly full of white men.

'I realised that the trauma experienced by the women I was working with needed a much more in-depth training, than even the social work training or an academic training, or even all the training you go on to be part of the women's movement.'

Despite how many women feel about Freud, and the 'white, Eurocentric, colonial, model' that psychoanalytic therapy still employs (Suryia's words), Freud's insights into human nature *are* still meaningful, as I learned from my own experience in therapy.

Suryia set up services which work at the intersection between rape and racism, and it wasn't easy. There were barriers, some subtle, others less so, such as not having the right kind of space to provide training. Now she works with a group called the Women of Colour Solidarity Space.

'And over again, what women of colour are saying is, it's very hard to call out racism when people are feminists and we're all supposed to be sisters together.'

There is still denial.

What *sustains* the women I have spoken to?

Lade Smith told me how she personally challenges the negative impact of racism such as she experienced from the delegate at the conference, 'You do your *own* cognitive therapy. I tell myself *you're a doctor!* I give myself all the positive reinforcement that I can.'

Elena, grieving for her mother, told me how she found non-judgemental peer support and sisterhood in an organisation for Black women.

'Being able to share your lived experience with other like-minded individuals across the diaspora of Black women was so important to me.'

Suryia Nayak said the things that have sustained her are her networks of women, both those working at the grassroots and in institutions, and her knowledge. When I asked her, 'What needs to change?' she told me how sometimes people working in services have to step back from their everyday battles and revisit history. She pointed to the wall of books that framed one side of our Zoom call:

> I know that if I don't dip into one of them, and most of them are Black feminist books, I get to feel ill.
>
> There's this thing called *historical amnesia*, which Audre Lorde talks about,[35] where we disconnect from the wisdom, the nourishment and the richness of all the documented struggles.
>
> Nothing's new under the sun.

What Must Change?

First our society needs to acknowledge there is a problem.

There is still denial in the media.[36] Denial that a privileged white woman asking a Black woman at an event at Buckingham Palace, 'Where are you from?' might even have the potential to be perceived as racist.

Researching and writing this chapter has reminded me personally of the times I could have not only offered more support to colleagues at work who were victims of racism but been more of a true ally by challenging those who abused and bullied them. My *own* fear of bullies prevented me from doing that.

But I should have done more.

We all must.

Especially white feminists who ignored the problems of Black women for decades, and still do.

When it comes to mental health care, 'Just an *acknowledgement* that we are not all the same would help,' Elena told me.

Being 'colour blind' doesn't work any better than being 'gender neutral'.

No surprise there.

The psychiatrist Suman Fernando talks about how psychiatric and psychological power coalesce with racism[37] to jointly oppress. But for women it is more complex still, because gender and race intersect in such a way that Black and ethnic minoritised women are not only sometimes afraid of seeking help from mental care, but they are *invisible* to services and their needs are ignored.

I've learned how necessary it is for mental health services to collaborate with non-governmental organisations that are trusted by the women in communities and run by them. Too often they are ignored, underfunded or even have to fight for their own survival, as Southall Black Sisters had to with Ealing Council in London. They proposed a single domestic violence service for the community on the grounds of 'equality' and 'cohesion', in other words to *promote* inequality once more.[38]

Southall Black Sisters received tremendous support from the community.

The council lost.

Dawn Edge said she didn't know any Black person to whom she would have to explain about being followed around at the shops. But she's had to explain it to me, and many others like me. Those of us who have attended 'cultural competence training', but still operate on our autopilots in our everyday work, instead of reflecting on what we've learned.

Mental health care *must* take on board discrimination and racism, in both how we train our staff and how we design and run our services. It is a key part of the 'social' bit of the 'biopsychosocial' approach, paying attention to physical, psychological and social aspects of a person's care, that we psychiatrists always talk about but often fail to fully put into practice.

It's time for some action.

Stop writing reports on it and *start really making a difference.*

But remembering how *gender* matters *too.*

When I saw Nina Simone perform in the late 1980s, I didn't realise she received none of the royalties from her big hit 'My Baby Just Cares for Me', made popular by a television commercial for Chanel perfume. As a young, Black, woman performer she had signed away the rights in 1958 before she even left the studio.

With the help of an attorney, she filed several lawsuits, resulting in the largest sum ever achieved for a 'reuse' fee for a recording.[39]

Just days before her death in 2003, the Curtis Institute of Music, who turned her down decades earlier, finally awarded her an honorary degree.

Too damned late.

7

● ● ● ● ● ●

Where Gender, Sex and Mental Health Collide

In 1960, a former merchant seaman from Liverpool called George Jamieson underwent a pioneering operation in Casablanca. The last words that the surgeon Dr Georges Burou said to him before the anaesthetic were, 'Bonjour Monsieur'. Seven hours later, he greeted him once more with, 'Bonjour Mademoiselle'.[1]

April Ashley, only the second British citizen to have a sex-change operation, had arrived.

As a young teenager I learned about April Ashley's transition by reading the tabloid newspapers that came into our home every day. I didn't understand then how much the press was and is still responsible for much of the vile stigma and harm experienced by people who don't fit society's norms. They not only 'outed' April Ashley, who was by 1961 a successful model,[2] but reported in salacious detail the sad story of how she was denied a divorce by a judge in 1970 from an aristocrat, because she was 'not a woman for the purpose of marriage, but a biological male, and has been so since birth'.[3]

She had never been legally married.

How much have our attitudes to sex and gender really changed since then?

'Glad to be Gay'

The distinctions between sexuality and gender were clarified about a century ago by the very same pioneering doctor and sexologist, Magnus Hirschfeld, who helped Lili Elbe, the trans woman played by Eddie Redmayne in *The Danish Girl* (who was, as an aside, coached by April Ashley). To help, there is a saying that 'sexual orientation is who you go to bed *with*, and gender is who you go to bed *as*'.

Some attitudes *have* changed in the last 40 years.

In 1979, as Tom Robinson sang his anthem 'Glad to be Gay', AIDS (Acquired Immune Deficiency Syndrome), for which homosexual men were to be blamed by the tabloid press, was only just over the horizon. Less than a decade later in 1987, Margaret Thatcher told the Conservative Party conference: 'Children are being taught they have an inalienable right to be gay. All of those children are being cheated of a sound start in life.'[4]

It was in this context that a close colleague admonished me out of the blue. The previous evening, as she was leaving the office, I had asked her to pass on my best wishes to her female partner. It was just second nature to me to think of her and her partner as a couple, but I failed to appreciate the context in which gay and lesbian people were then living. This anxiety about being 'outed' as lesbian, even though male homosexuality had in fact been legal in England and Wales since 1967, and female homosexuality had never been against the law, would be further reinforced by the infamous Section 28 of the

Local Government Act 1988, which prohibited the 'promotion of homosexuality' by local authorities.

The American Psychiatric Association voted to remove homosexuality from its diagnostic manual in 1973[5] so that it would no longer be considered a 'psychiatric disorder'. But before that time, electroshock 'treatments' were given, not only for men but also, as recent research[6] carried out by Hel Spandler and Sarah Carr has revealed, for women.

Hel, a professor of mental health who has edited *Asylum* magazine for many years, told me more about it:

> There was very little known about lesbians and the mental health system. Men were *offered* aversion therapy, and if they didn't accept, they'd have gone to prison. Women's homosexuality wasn't any more accepted than men's. But it wasn't *criminalised*. Or rather, it was maybe *indirectly* criminalised in the sense that because lesbians weren't accepted or visible, they tended to be driven underground. I think maybe a lot of poor or working-class lesbians in the 40s and 50s ended up either in sex work, on the streets, or with drug and alcohol problems and sometimes ended up in prison. So, we never heard about *women* having aversion therapy. Yet aversion therapy was given to some women, including trans women, from the early 1960s through to the 1970s.

Hel, with Sarah Carr, identified 10 examples of young lesbian and bisexual women receiving aversion therapy in England, which, from the description of one who later wrote an essay about it, involved receiving electric shocks when pictures of women came up on the screen. This woman received this 'treatment' at Crumpsall Hospital in North Manchester (where, a generation later, I studied psychiatry). She volunteered to have it. It 'put her off' women but only for a while and it didn't make her like men. It made her feel ashamed, and she later went on to have satisfying relationships with women.

More than 50 years later, in the *Psychologist* magazine,[7] she described how, while doing a Master's degree in Women's Studies during the 1980s:

> For the first time, I saw with great clarity the meaning of the physical violence and the emotional violence that had been committed against

me. The tears I wept helped to heal the damage. Other healing came from the feminist theory and knowledge that helped me to join up the fragments that until that point had not made much sense.

A few other women were given aversion therapy against their will, but with their parents' permission, because they were 'under the age of consent', even though there *wasn't* an age of consent for sex between women at that time. One eventually married a man, but others describe the treatment as 'unsuccessful', and they were still attracted to women.

The 'therapy', mostly delivered by psychologists and nurses, some of whom were women, and overseen by (male) psychiatrists, was abhorrent.

There were positive accounts too, of lesbian women's experiences of psychology and psychiatry during the post-Second World War period, where women were reassured that their sexuality wasn't pathological and didn't need 'treatment', but it's painful to read how *acceptable* it apparently was to attempt to 'treat' lesbian women in the recent past. To rid them of their supposed deviance.

It is extraordinary how out of touch those mental health professionals were with the changes that were happening in society, at the very time they were carrying this out.

And by the early 1980s, radical lesbian feminists not only viewed heterosexuality as something that should be overthrown but also were *very* critical of psychiatry, viewing it not only as patriarchal but extremely harmful to women.[8]

So, what is *still* happening in those places where we look back at the past and say, 'Well it was all different then wasn't it?'

What has and hasn't changed?

Across the world there are still countries where homosexuality is illegal and even potentially a capital offence.

Many people are also still subjected to conversion 'therapy' where efforts are made to change a person's sexual orientation or gender identity, with 5% of LGBT people reporting being pressured to seek this, rising to 9% of those from BAME backgrounds.[9]

Stonewall, the UK-based LBGTQ+ rights charity, also found that 60% of lesbians and 72% of those identifying as bi women had experienced anxiety in the previous year and 37% of lesbians and 50% of bi women had felt that life was not worth living. Experience of virulent homophobia, discrimination, a sense of social isolation and hate crimes contributed to this, such as the vicious attack on two women which took place on a London bus in 2019, because they refused an order from their goading male persecutors to kiss each other.[10]

Health care was criticised too, for its ignorance. One participant commented how, 'Medical professionals are not that good with lesbians. I don't go to the GP that often because they are not that familiar with lesbian issues usually.'

But particularly worrying for me as a psychiatrist is the use of uncertainty or ambivalence around issues of gender and sexuality to label people with another diagnosis, 'borderline personality disorder'. Mal, who identifies as non-binary and was given this diagnosis at the age of 18 said:

> I remember, in my notes, mentioning the way that I dressed as being androgynous, and then that being seen as like evidence of an 'unstable sense of self'. There is a time where it mentioned that I came in a dress. And then in another appointment, I was wearing trousers and a shirt. It does feel like mental health services still have this very outdated view of sexuality and gender.

Something other folk mentioned too: a requirement to conform to stereotypes.

If people who identify as lesbian, bi, queer or non-binary are facing problems in mental health services, what about *transgender* health care and in particular the problems faced by trans women?

The Struggles of Trans Women

Reflecting on my question about trans women's mental health problems, an old GP colleague who has spent much of his career working with trans women said to me, 'If society accepted that trans women *were* women, I don't think they would have any more nor I suppose any less mental health problems than women in general.'

I've borne that reply in mind ever since.

I first met Sameera, an anaesthetist in her forties now working in London, when she spoke at a conference about her experiences as a transgender woman, growing up in India, and then immigrating to the UK.

Sameera told me how she distinctly remembers what happened when as 4-year-old Sameer, as she then was, she wandered into the bathroom without thinking when a young female relative came to stay. 'That was the start of contrasting why my body was different.'

Having spent her early years exclusively with girls, from whom she had not felt in any way distinct, Sameer found it very difficult to relate to boys when she moved to an all-boys middle school.

'I was very feminised. Boys started bullying me. Pinching me on my buttocks. Saying "get away, get away, get away. You can't be with me. You can't sit next to me." And that had a very negative impact on me.'

Inside she was *utterly* confused: 'I knew I was a girl.' But her family were pushing her to behave in a more stereotyped masculine way: 'Be like a man.'

Isolating herself, her studies initially began to suffer. However, she then found that being alone enabled her to focus even more on her goal of studying medicine. A chance opportunity to be involved in a drama introduced her to dancing, forbidden to muslim boys, and she would secretly cross-dress at home alone, and *dance*.

'I used to love to dance it was like an expression of me, that girl inside me.'

At university she discovered that the out-of-date, homophobic and transphobic, medical literature far from eased her anxiety and huge sense of guilt ('Why am I like this?'), which she tried to assuage through prayer. But by discovering a different world via the internet, and through reading modern psychotherapy texts, she began slowly to accept herself. Having avoided her parents' hopes for marriage by moving to the south of India, she was finally able to tell her father that she was attracted to men, though not about her internal feelings that 'there was a woman inside me'.

And she did achieve happiness in a relationship with a man during which the woman inside 'used to come out whenever we were together'.

Over a period of eight years, Sameer was treated by an endocrinologist and then finally underwent gender reassignment surgery.

Becoming Sameera.

Sameera's trans identity was socially accepted in southern India where Tamils readily accept non-binary genders. *Kothis* describe themselves in Tamil as *pen manaam konda aan* ('a woman's heart in a man's body'[11]) and in India it was legally possible for Sameera to be recognised as 'transgender' rather than simply male or female.

'I had liberty to identify myself as the way I am. I wasn't boxed. And when you're not in a box, you have such a huge amount of freedom.'

Sameera's words echo the *liberation* that the writer Jan Morris talked about wanting in her memoir *Conundrum*, when she finally began her journey to becoming a woman.[12]

Sameera arrived in the UK during the pandemic to begin work in the NHS. However, when registering with the General Medical Council, there were only two choices for gender: male and female.

She told me how she now felt that she was now being *pushed* towards identifying as a woman.

'I'm a different person. Why can't you acknowledge the difference on paper – that different people do exist?'

Much of the emotional distress that trans women experience in the UK is because of the *enormous* delay in the UK before getting access to gender identity services, with little support during which time the kind of mental health problems that Sameera described can get worse.

But what happens in society also matters a great deal too.

Dr Cleo Madeleine, an independent researcher who works with the organisation Gendered Intelligence, explained the impact of political pressure, amplified by the mainstream media and right-wing press with misinformation, *particularly* on trans women's mental health, and an awful *acceptance* that anti-trans sentiment can be expressed publicly and loudly.

'The extent and the negativity of the coverage, particularly since Covid, exacerbates a sense of isolation and often feeds into a sense of paranoia . . . with the idea that public services aren't appropriate for trans people and their participation in public life is *dangerous or unwanted.*'

Cleo described it as a 'climate of fear'.

Dr James Barrett, head of the adult Gender Identity Service in London, put it succinctly:

It's everybody feeling that they are at liberty to inquire about the arrangement of your genitals or assume that you're going to be some kind of rapist.

Just blatant nonsense being spoken about you, as if you're not a kind of a proper person and that you *can* be talked about in that way.

In her superbly well-argued book *The Transgender Issue: An Argument for Justice*, Shon Faye, a trans woman, tells how Britain is having a *deafening* conversation about trans people now, but the 'wrong conversation'. Trans people have become an *issue*. But no one wants to talk about the challenges facing them, only 'their issues with us'.[13]

And the problems they face are many.

The Stonewall survey[14] found that 46% of trans people had considered taking their own life in the previous year and 67% had experienced depression, much of this related to the fear, abuse and even violence they experience.

I asked James Barrett about rate of suicide, *not* the same as having suicidal thoughts. Is it higher for trans people?

'Yes. And no. It is before people hit treatment, but the suicide rate of patients who are in treatment is about the population average.'

So, getting access quickly is important, but difficult. And how early should 'early' be?

'The number of referrals has doubled every year since 1966.'

Shon Faye[15] also highlights how intersectionality is crucial to understanding the extent of the problems facing trans people. They particularly experience bullying at school, family rejection, homelessness, domestic violence and discrimination. Black and ethnic minoritised trans people and other marginalised people, such as those who are disabled and refugees, will be *even more likely* to face all of these.

The wait to be seen at one of the UK's seven gender identity clinics can be anything between two and five years depending on where you live. And it's difficult to access any appropriate mental health support before the clinic assessment, or services such as speech and language therapy to help with your voice or laser treatment for facial hair, without paying for private therapy – which, inevitably, some do to avoid the wait. Trans health care is about so much more than hormones and genital surgery (which in the UK 60% of trans women will undergo[16]).

Until recently, a predominantly male workforce of psychiatrists and psychologists have been the 'gatekeepers' to trans health care in the UK, and, according to Harry Josephine Giles, the award-winning Scottish poet, trans women's memoirs and advice booklets tell frequent stories of being refused treatment because they weren't wearing feminine enough clothing.[17] Trans women are subject to misogyny too and expected to conform to gender norms.

The system can be harsh and brutal.

But perhaps not as extraordinary as in the 1960s, when the founding psychiatrist of the transgender service in London, Dr John Randell, gave evidence *for* April Ashley's husband in the divorce court that she was in fact a 'homosexual transexual male'.

That must have caused her terrible distress.

This gatekeeping by psychiatry and the need for a diagnosis doesn't exist in 20 other countries around the world, and there have been attempts in Scotland, where I live, to make it easier to *self*-identify without any medical assessment and to acquire a gender identity certificate after three months of living in your chosen gender.

Opposing views on this were provided to legislators by two different United Nations experts.

Victor Madrigal-Borloz, the UN's independent expert on protection against violence and discrimination based on sexual orientation and gender identity, argued that the evidence from other countries where self-identification is standard does *not* support fears about abuse of the system by predatory males.[18]

However, the UN special rapporteur on violence against women and girls, Reem Alsalem, said it 'would potentially open the door for violent males who identify as men to abuse the process of acquiring a gender certificate and the rights that are associated with it'.[19]

Legislation to approve self-identification was passed in the devolved Scottish Parliament after campaigning by trans rights activists with support from many feminists. 'Gender critical' feminists, now the favoured pre-fix for feminists who question trans inclusion, firmly believe that sex cannot be changed and campaigned vigorously against it.

It was, however, blocked by the UK government.

Between feminists, the fight over trans inclusion has been going on for a very long time with vigorous opposition from some such as Janice Raymond, a lesbian radical feminist in the 1970s and, in more recent years, veteran second-wave feminists such as Germaine Greer. However, for Shulamith Firestone, writing in 1970, the end goal of feminist revolution was to be the elimination of the sex *distinction* itself: so that genital differences between human beings would no longer matter.[20]

Andrea Dworkin, the radical feminist icon, supported this utopian view strongly, and her partner, John Stoltenberg, has written how Dworkin was a true trans-ally, and did not support in any way the 'biological essentialism' of the 'gender critical' feminists' anti-trans stance: 'Andrea absolutely *did* know, as a woman and as a Jew, what biologically essentialist scapegoating looks and feels like.'[21] Recently, Catherine MacKinnon, a veteran feminist influenced by Dworkin, has powerfully criticised the transmisogyny of gender critical feminism and its unwillingness to accept transfeminism.[22]

Whatever your view, it's not difficult to see how repeated denial of the lived experience of trans people is causing real psychological harm. Trans women are regularly and unhelpfully called 'men' by gender critical feminists.

Sameera told me that *all* the discrimination that she has experienced in her job as an anaesthetist has been from women, and it has been very distressing.

There have also been linkups between gender critical feminist groups in the USA and right-wing organisations with a similar anti-trans agenda; organisations that *also* oppose abortion and same-sex marriage.[23]

Interesting bedfellows for feminists.

Meanwhile, the toxic media attention in society has not only been on, usually older, trans women but also directed at much younger people, either assigned female at birth (AFAB) or 'natal females' – the language you use tends to vary with your opinion – now identifying as male.

What is happening to them?

Girls Will Be Boys

There are some things in life where opinions differ so much that even published 'evidence' gets interpreted in different ways, either supporting or negating your opinions, depending on what point of view you hold and which 'side' you take. Antidepressant research is one of these. Gender dysphoria is another.

What is *absolutely clear* from the independent investigation carried out by Hilary Cass,[24] a paediatrician who has carried out a review of Gender Identity Development Service (GIDS) in London (which serves the whole of the UK except Scotland) is that there has been a considerable increase in the number of young people, but especially teenage AFABs, being referred for 'gender dysphoria' (the diagnostic term from DSM 5).

In 2009, there were 39 adolescents (15 AFAB) and 12 children (2 AFAB). By 2016 this had risen to a total of 1,497 adolescents (1,071 AFAB) and 269 children (131 AFAB) referred to GIDS in the UK. The *steepest* increase was in 2014–15 and in 2020 there were around 2,500 referrals a year and a waiting time of more than two years.

For many years the approach was to offer assessment and support and provide treatment to block puberty when children reach maturity, at about age 15, with oestrogen or testosterone only being given to feminise or masculinise at age 16. But research carried out in Amsterdam[25] suggested that puberty blockers would be better given in the *early* stages of puberty, to give young people more time to explore their gender identity free from the distress caused by secondary sex characteristics such as breasts and body hair developing. In 2011, the UK services adopted this new 'Dutch' protocol, as did other countries, with earlier use of puberty blockers. Feminising/masculinising hormones were started age 16 and surgery was allowed at 18 in the UK (in the USA it is available, in some places, at an earlier age, although religious groups and conservative politicians are up in arms about it[26]).

Meanwhile some working in the service became increasingly concerned about the change in those coming to the clinics, now with a marked majority of young people AFAB, but with increasingly complex mental health problems too. Other countries were experiencing this shift as well. There was concern about something called 'rapid onset gender dysphoria' in young girls in online chat rooms perhaps reinforcing their self-diagnosis of being trans.[27] Then, after two women, including Keira Bell who had 'de-transitioned', took the Tavistock Hospital Trust to court, there was a ruling that children under 16 were unlikely to be mature enough to give informed consent to receiving puberty blockers. Even though that decision *was* overturned on appeal, the process was set in motion to review of the system.

I've spoken to people who interpret the huge increase in AFAB adolescents coming to the gender identity development service in very different ways.

Dr James Barrett, head of the Adult Gender Identity Service told me:

> I think the reason people didn't present before was they could more or less contain their stresses socially. But *now*, it's probably people realising that they don't *have* to live in a particular way. I don't think this is any commoner. And the clue is that with increased numbers the mean age has progressively fallen. It's the *same people* speaking up earlier.

Finn Mackay, who identifies as non-binary, has talked about how they considered transition in the past but decided against it, having come to terms with their 'in-between' state.[28] Finn does describe in *Female Masculinities*[29] how some 'butch' lesbians (sometimes called 'masculine lesbians') they interviewed for their own research had felt under pressure to transition to men. Nevertheless, Finn is critical of those who think the experience of trans men is merely a flight from our misogynist society, or that they are 'victims being led astray by trans culture'.[30]

Cleo Madeleine certainly thinks there's a sense in which young trans men or young trans masculine people are treated in the media and the public eye as from a patriarchal perspective: 'Girls, who have ruined or harmed their bodies.'

From the opposing perspective, Dr Anna Hutchinson, one of the psychologists who resigned from the Tavistock GIDS service because they were worried about young people progressing too rapidly to hormone treatment, has expressed serious concerns about the rise in young AFAB coming for help in recent years,[31] and what then happens to them:

> Initially it was thought, 'Okay, well, this is a balancing out. If this is a phenomenon that has been in the human population forever there'll be as many females as there are males', but in about 2012, the number

of females coming forward for help overtook the number of males. And this was an *entirely different* demographic.

There always have been a high number of autistic people who experience gender dysphoria, up to 50% in some services, in both adults and children.

But the new group of 'natal females' coming for help had more complex additional mental health problems than ever before, including early trauma, eating disorders, domestic violence and having been in care, now called 'looked after children'.

'And I guess the numbers increased so profoundly, that the psychological complexity couldn't really be denied.'

This has developed into one of the most political topics in health care with the suggestion that young people who identify as trans are at risk of being denied the right of self-determination, and those critical of what has been happening called 'transphobic'. I'm aware I'm risking that by even mentioning it here.

'But in the middle of this,' Anna continued, 'you've got this large number of natal females or AFAB (whatever terminology you use it's wrong!) identifying as male and coming forward for help *in great distress.*'

Anna says the data from historical studies suggests a natural resolution of gender dysphoria in 80–90% of cases in children, but with early affirmation and medical treatment there is now about 99–100% persistence.[32]

And then there are those who 'detransition'. Those whom Anna works with were all natal females who have taken the decision to revert to their original gender. She says that, if their problems seemed complex before they are even more so afterwards.

So, the discussion about 'What is best?' has become a binary choice between the practice of affirming a young person in their preferred gender and starting medication or starting psychotherapy. Anna insists we mustn't mix up offering talking therapy to help people become more comfortable with their bodies and to provide more choice in treatment with trying to argue someone *out* of identifying as transgender.

But no one can or should be *forced* to undergo therapy.

That is abusive.

What they may benefit from, however, is time, and space, to talk about what has been happening in their lives.

And, as an outsider to this debate, I do wonder why *everything* must be a binary choice? Why can't *both* explanations for the increase in AFAB or 'natal females' have a part to play in explaining this increase? Why does it *have* to be one or the other?

Do we really know enough what is happening yet? I don't think we do. *Much* more research is needed.

From beginning to research this book, and hearing about the increasing distress and mental health problems in young women in their teens in Chapter 1, I've been concerned about what is happening to young women in our society.

We all should be.

Perhaps *some* of these may be seeking answers to their problems in their gender identity *and* focusing down on medical solutions without being given other options?

I'm also reminded of what I know about the dissatisfaction with body image young women with eating disorders experience and there is a recognised connection between gender dysphoria and eating disorders.[33]

The Cass Review in the UK says that 'Children and young people with gender incongruence or dysphoria must receive the same standards of clinical care, assessment and treatment as every other child or young person accessing health services.' It also says there shouldn't be an 'unquestioning' gender affirmative approach with children and young people, and we still have much to learn about the safety and longer-term outcomes of the treatments being offered, particularly puberty blockers. There isn't enough research into this, and what there is tends to be interpreted according to ideological standpoints. As a result, puberty blockers will only be provided with enrolment into a research study.[34]

This remains completely unacceptable to many trans people.

What seems clear is we *mustn't* prevent young AFAB people for whom the decision to transition is clearly the right one, who understand the potential consequences in terms of their physical health and future fertility of having hormone treatment and are able to consent, from going ahead with it.

Getting this right is going to be difficult. Even harder if we avoid talking about it.

And it has ended up as one of several battlegrounds in the 'gender wars' in which what I hear from both 'sides' are expressions of fear, rage and even cynicism that the other 'side' is willing to listen to them at all.

None of this is good for the mental health of the trans women and men who find themselves at the centre of this – whose *very existence* seems, to them, to be up for public debate.

What Must Change?

'I think the whole conversation around transgender issues needs the heat and the smoke taking out of it.'

I couldn't agree more with Cleo Madeleine.

The current atmosphere is vicious and lacking in mutual respect.

Constant misgendering of non-binary and trans people causes distress. But publicly raising concerns about the impact of gender self-identification on *women* can lead to accusations of transphobia too.

When it comes to the current war being fought over self-identification, there is something else that must be considered. Not only an epidemic but also a very tangible *fear* of male violence which affects *all* of us, women, men, and trans people too. This is the context for what Finn Mackay also a radical *trans-inclusive* feminist, calls women's fears and defensiveness about people they assume to be men sharing their intimate spaces.[35]

As I psychiatrist, I treated women (and men) with post-traumatic symptoms who could not be alone in a room with a man because of their previous experiences of abuse. Women who found being on a mixed sex ward with men utterly terrifying.

'You can't forget a lifetime of conditioning,' said Finn.

None of us can. This is how women are raised.

To 'stay safe'.

We are going to continue to need access to 'women only' spaces, but that will require much consideration of how they are defined. Biological reductionism would have excluded April Ashley who lived her life, like so many other trans women, in every way as a woman. Policing of 'gender conformity' is unacceptable too. Yet our politicians are now talking about 'safe spaces for biological women'.

Really? It's just not that simple.

So, I *can* understand both the distress of trans people who feel frustrated and angry at having to jump through the hoops of psychiatric assessment and being blamed for something that is *not* to do with them – violence from which they are also at risk – *and* the distress and fear of women at losing their safe spaces.

Feminists and activists need to work hard at finding ways of hearing and accommodating *both* points of view, rather than constantly battling with each other. Being able to listen to, understand and empathise, if not agree, with each other is crucial to finding a way forward.

It's something I've learned from years of psychotherapy.

Meanwhile, almost no attention is given to the needs of trans men in all this debate, other than changing the language used in maternity and gynaecological care. This has alienated many women, and caused some concern for those whose first language isn't English.

We must find ways to ensure that *everyone* feels welcomed.

The same applies to domestic violence and rape crisis services.

'Young masculine identified young people,' said Finn, 'may have more male friends and they think that their risk is lower. They don't see themselves as being a target for that type of violence.' And they may not be comfortable with the term 'female' or at all pleased to be misgendered.

It's disrespectful.

Like all people subject to intersectional inequalities, LGBTQ+ people who are at risk need allies among us.

That's a role we must all play.

We need to recognise that many of us are still on a *journey* with our own sexuality and gender.

As Sameera's story demonstrates, 'absolutes' don't reflect real lives.

People who work in services need to reach out to LGBTQ+ community organisations too.

This can be as little as, if you run a drop-in service, simply putting a pride flag in the window, or as much as even collaborating on community health projects and befriending schemes to combat isolation and ensuring all your staff are trained to work with the LGBTQ+ community.

In 2017, the Royal College of Psychiatrists issued an apology for the harm done to lesbian, gay and bisexual people with 'conversion therapies' in the past, and today it 'considers that interventions that claim to convert transgender and gender-diverse people into cisgender people are without scientific foundation and thus both unethical and unacceptable'.[36]

However, the British government has yet to ban it or indeed any kind of LGBTQ+ 'conversion therapy'.

That's unacceptable.

April Ashley finally obtained a birth certificate recognising her as female in 2005, with the support of Labour deputy prime minister John Prescott, who, decades before, had once rented a room in the same boarding house as her. The UK Gender Recognition Act, for which she campaigned, was passed into law in 2004.

In a recent documentary[37] Boy George said of her, '*It wasn't drag.* 'April was a woman.'

She died aged 86 in 2021.

8
• • • • • •

Survivors of Male Violence

I met this guy.

He was *real* nice.

We got married. He was working and everything. And then after we got married, it just went downhill. He beat me up all the time. I remember one time specifically. He put a gun in my mouth and said he was going to kill me.

The neighbour called the cops, and they came ... but he was standing behind the door with a gun. So, they left.

I was bleeding. But they left.

My parents said 'You're married. You need to work it out.' And I really didn't have anywhere to go. It was my apartment we'd moved into. And he was just emptying my bank account. I found out later he was doing a lot of cocaine.

I just felt like I was between a rock and a hard place.

When I was trying to contact survivors of male violence who were willing to tell me what happened to them, Susan, who is now 65, got in touch with me about what she went through 40 years ago in rural America.

She recounted it as though it was only yesterday. Still fresh in her mind.

'I didn't have anywhere to go.'

Some things, at least, have changed. Or have they?

The risk that women face from male violence is *acknowledged*. But what are we doing about it?

Thousands of miles away in Chiswick, London, and 14 years before Susan's violent marriage began, Erin Pizzey founded the first women's' refuge in England. Her book, *Scream Quietly or the Neighbours Will Hear*,[1] has been sitting on my bookshelf since I was a medical student.

I didn't grow up in a household where there was physical violence between my parents. My mother told me once that if Dad *ever* hit her, he already knew that she would leave him. He had an explosive temper. However, *both* of my parents hit me in anger – my father very hard indeed at times. I've never been hit by any other man, but I recognised something personal in the deep sense of shame that abused women told me about – of feeling disgraced and wanting to hide.

I used to run away and stay in my room for hours.

The house in Chiswick was the start of a movement, the UK charity Refuge. It now supports tens of thousands of women and children each year. Women can, and do, escape to somewhere safe, where they can be supported and helped to rebuild their lives.

However, Refuge, and the other main organisation, Women's Aid, must still turn many away who they are simply unable to help through lack of resources.[2]

And the violence just goes on, and on.

The Most Dangerous Place

In her book, *Eve Was Framed*, about how the justice system fails women, campaigning barrister Helena Kennedy said that the home, as Susan discovered, is by far the most dangerous place for a woman.[3]

'I never planned to research domestic violence,' the perinatal mental illness and domestic violence expert Professor Louise Howard told me when we met online.

During her extensive research with pregnant women in the 1990s, she heard how they were regularly asked about experience of child abuse but *not* about violence in current or recent relationships.

'They were so full of shame and embarrassment, and very scared about what would be the result of disclosing. Would that mean that their children would be removed because they weren't protecting them from this perpetrator?'

Like me, she hadn't been trained at all in how to ask about domestic violence, but she began to ask more about relationships in her clinic once she had learnt how to ask and safely respond:

I was sometimes shocked by my own unconscious biases around class . . . We're talking about an event like a professional woman being pinned against the wall, and somebody's trying to strangle them. I never expected that kind of disclosure.

Being a woman in those clinics and also being a woman researcher, made me much more able to listen to those voices.

WHO estimates that about 30% of women worldwide have been subjected to either physical or sexual intimate partner violence (IPV) in their lifetimes[4] and a quarter of women aged 15–49 years who have been in a relationship have experienced this at least once in their lifetime.

Its utterly shocking that women in the USA are *more* likely to be murdered during pregnancy or soon after childbirth than to die from the three leading obstetric causes of maternal mortality: hypertensive disorders, haemorrhage, or sepsis.[5]

Liz, now 54, has spent most of her life living with the consequences of domestic abuse, both emotional and physical. She remembers her early life as very happy, until, at the age of 12, she discovered her father was having an affair and innocently told her grandmother, resulting in appalling rejection by her father who began to tell her she was ugly and worthless.

'We were all sitting around the table chatting and then my dad just stopped eating and put his knife and fork down, very calmly. He looked at me, went nose to nose and said, "You disgust me. You're filthy, you're dirty, go away."'

So, as soon as she could, she left.

She was introduced to a man who was then in prison.

'He was going to be the one *regardless* of his crime. I needed someone who showed me some love. He got out of prison and then after six months I became his punch bag.'

Liz's life became tightly *controlled* by her partner. He cut her off from friends and family, insisting they both work at the same supermarket. She had to sit alone while he flirted with other women but then interrogated her about who she had been with if she missed the bus home and arrived late. She had to pay for all the household expenses out of her meagre allowance, which meant they rapidly got into debt.

This, she was told, was her fault.

He slammed the car brakes on while she was pregnant to see if she would miscarry and beat her while she was heavily pregnant with their second child. At the hospital she spoke to the police but then declined to press charges.

'And then I had him back . . . because I loved him.'

She was visibly distressed while we spoke, even though this was 30 years ago. I asked her if she hoped he would change.

'Yeah, it was alright for a bit. Then it all started again.'

She eventually managed to get away from him, but he would still come around and harass her, sometimes pinning her into a chair.

'I couldn't get out. Even now, I don't like people standing in doorways. My stepson, when he used to come around, he used to take his top off and stand in the doorway with his arms up on the side of the door.

'I can't deal with that. Because *I can't get out.*'

She rarely sits in a room with the door closed. I could hear, in her trembling voice, how that utter terror of male violence has persisted over decades.

Not Only Physical but Also Psychological Harm

I met many women like Liz throughout my career, from my time in the Emergency Department through to the psychiatric clinic.

The sense of shame women experience can be overwhelming.[6]

Shame is different from guilt. You can feel guilty for things that you have done, but shame is about how the world sees you and your own core sense of self-worth. You want to hide away and disappear.

Jo, who has worked with Women's Aid for several years, told me how the ethos of her work was to provide 'unconditional positive regard'.

'Because we find that's most effective in reducing shame. Shame about judgements from others. "I went back to him, so I've asked for it." Shame about what everyone's saying about it. Shame about using alcohol to try and cope with it when I'm not supposed to.'

Shame can mean that you don't tell others about what is happening to you and try to conceal it. You normalise it and minimise it.

You blame yourself.

If you've experienced abuse in childhood, such as Liz, or witnessed IPV, that increases your risk of intimate partner violence as an adult. Together these can increase your chance of having mental health problems as an adult. As I learned from my own experience both as a practitioner and as a patient, damage caused by what parents do, and fail to do, can work to prevent women from making effective and safe relationships as adults.

Mental health problems are *not* an inevitable consequence of IPV but anxiety, depression, post-traumatic stress disorder, psychosis, self-harm, substance misuse *and* getting a diagnosis of borderline personality disorder (BPD) are all more common in people who have experienced IPV than those who haven't, and they are more likely to have *persistent* mental health problems.[7]

Liz has been on antidepressants for most of her life, but with little benefit. Cognitive behaviour therapy didn't help much either.

So, a holistic approach to helping women is crucial. Providing advice, advocacy and legal support, access to counselling and psychological therapy, and ongoing support which is often in groups. Specific psychiatric diagnosis and treatment may be needed; for example, when depression and anxiety doesn't improve or becomes more severe, or for post-traumatic stress disorder which requires *specific* psychological therapy. But getting access to these therapies can be hard.

Jessica Taylor, feminist author of *Sexy but Psycho*,[8] argues that a woman's diagnostic label can detract from the real and horrific trauma she has suffered. She and her diagnosis then become the 'problem' for society, sometimes even more than the man who subjected her to the violence in the first place.

I absolutely agree.

And in the legal system, pathologising victims, by calling them 'mentally ill', can mean that they are then seen as unreliable witnesses. A diagnosis of BPD can be particularly damaging. In the family court system, such 'evidence' is abusively used by violent men in custody and access battles with their ex-wives and partners.

But where I disagree with Jessica Taylor is that psychiatry is *always* harmful.

It isn't and should aim *never* to be.

But it does need to be *much better* at helping women who have experienced male violence.

'Women *do* get depressed,' said Dr Hannana Siddiqui at Southall Black Sisters, an organisation that works with women at risk of both domestic abuse and honour-based violence, 'and they do sometimes get clinically depressed. And a lot of the time it's not even diagnosed when it should have been. But I think where there has been a response from health services, it often becomes a kind of a medicalisation. The health service can fail to acknowledge the social problems.'

The woman becomes a *case of depression* rather than someone who is both depressed *and* subject to abuse and violence, which have played a key part in causing this. In my experience, failing to address *both* slows a woman's chance of recovery.

And one problem is that professionals may not only have received no training in IPV but also completely fail to understand the nature of coercive control.

Coercive Control

There are different kinds of intimate partner violence (physical, sexual, emotional, controlling behaviours), and you can distinguish between violence that is a reaction to anger or frustration and 'intimate terrorism' where violence is a way of reinforcing control. That control becomes pervasive with long-lasting psychological effects.

Freya survived many years of violent coercive control.

Her husband told her she was crazy, 'you're fucked up in the head, you're ruining our marriage', but when she sought help, he intercepted appointments from the counsellor she had started to see. As he began to lose control, she sensed he was becoming more physically dangerous:

I did think he was going to kill me.

I remember being in the kitchen on a phone to my solicitor and just looking at the window saying, 'Oh, my God, oh, my God, he's back. He's back. What am I going to do?' Really panicking. And I remember the solicitor laughing. I thought, 'Why are you laughing like, that. It's so risky because I'm *on the phone with someone*.'

I was terrified.

She discovered she had lost any sense of what 'reasonable' behaviour was. Writing a list for the solicitor of what had happened in her marriage, which included pushing her out in front of a car when she was five months pregnant, she was stunned by his reaction:

> People say, 'Why didn't she leave? Why didn't she just open the door and walk out when he's not there? When he's gone to work?' It would be *reasonable* to just open the door, wouldn't it? But they don't understand the way the control works. Someone doesn't have to be with you to have control over you. It operates over time and space.

There are many reasons why women don't leave.[9]

Coercive control, which Freya and Liz both described to me, is a key factor. The perpetrator makes the woman feel constantly afraid, usually with the threat of physical or sexual violence. The act of leaving can place her in *more* danger.

Then there are the practical barriers: finding housing, enough money to survive, care of the children and fear of losing them. There's also shame and guilt, including letting their own parents down, and even returning as Liz did at first, because of love.

Continued abuse traumatises and can prevent a woman from getting herself together to take the steps to leave. Particularly if they are still in hope that, one day, everything will work out. Women tell the doctor that the bruise on their face was caused by a fall. They may minimise the abuse, blame themselves once again and feel even more shame.

They get blamed by inept professionals for not leaving.

I have known situations where mental health professionals have failed to pick up on the pathological jealousy of a man who is checking on his wife's movements and only seen them together as a couple for a 'relationship problem', making disclosure impossible.

Pressurising women into having marital counselling can kill them.

When and if it finally comes to court, men can use the opportunity in the family courts to represent themselves as an *extension* of abuse and control. Continuing to try to abuse and control the woman within the courtroom. Meanwhile women who are trying to prevent their partners harming children if they are given access can be accused of 'parental alienation', but then get blamed if they do allow access and children are harmed.

It's impossible for them.

Freya finally left her husband at the beginning of a year.

'In the April after that, I remember bumping into someone I knew, I think it was a mum at school, in the supermarket and just chatting. And *all of a sudden*, I started to panic.'

She had been out for an hour. Her husband used to time her journeys. She was no longer with him, but she was *still* afraid.

She now has been diagnosed with severe, and yet *still* untreated, post-traumatic stress disorder. Flashbacks of being raped by him when she tried to leave him have led her to attempt suicide.

As Khatidja Chantler told me, when *repetition* of offences is considered,[10] 'in comparison to men, women are much more severely damaged and suffer the most serious consequences' from domestic violence.

But even this is challenged by some, both men and women.

Erin Pizzey, founder of the first refuge, later developed the theory that some women are *addicted* to violence and, when writer Helen Lewis tracked her down in her book *Difficult Women*,[11] she was working with an organisation which *denies* that domestic violence is a gendered problem.

It was so disappointing to discover that.

The pervasive and damaging impact of coercive control on a woman's psyche, the impact that Freya described, cannot be underestimated, but many still don't get it. Or want to.

When I first met Khatidja, she told me how a student had complained that the Duluth model[12] she was using to explain domestic violence was 'too feminist', despite it being globally accepted. Duluth, a town in Minnesota, has been at the forefront of innovative ways of reducing domestic violence in the community:

> I think what they were *wanting* me to say is that there are just as many female perpetrators of domestic abuse as there are male, and that's *just not the case*. Any evidence you look at will show the highly gendered nature of domestic abuse.
>
> But in our current study, we're looking at domestic homicide. And it's *women's bodies we are counting*.

Counting Dead Women

In January 2012, angered by the sheer volume of violent crimes against women, and discovering that the UK Office for National Statistics *only* records the sex of those who have been killed but not of the person who killed them, Karen Ingala Smith began a project: Counting Dead Women. She recorded female deaths at the hands of men contemporaneously,[13] and according to the subsequent Femicide Census[14] she developed, the number of women killed by men hovers between 124 and 168 per year, and on average 62% of these were killed by a current or former partner.

But this doesn't tell the whole story.

Domestic violence drives women to suicide. Women die to 'protect the family honour'. Women are killed in 'murder-suicides' by partners who cannot let a woman continue to live her own life.

A 2004 study[15] estimated that 1 in 8 of all female suicides and suicide attempts are related to domestic violence and abuse.

In 2013, Karen Blatchford started to count women who had taken their own lives after experiencing male violence. She records each woman on her twitter feed @we_are_nina (not invisible, not alone), but these deaths are not included in officially collected data. There are real problems in counting them accurately.

Karen told me, 'Our data are *so* poor. Currently we don't even record ethnicity.'

Coroners can now conclude unlawful killing and suicide 'on the balance of probabilities', and police have proposed that the legislation brought into law in the UK for coercive control in 2015 could be used against perpetrators in domestic abuse related suicide, but the maximum penalty is only five years. In France, if domestic abuse is a factor in a suicide, they can expect a sentence of up to 10 years and a fine of €150,000.[16]

Coroners can only go on the information they are given and will only know of the abuse if the police know, which they often don't, although domestic homicide reviews are now taking place after suicide where domestic abuse might be a factor.

Some 12 to 15 women are still dying in 'honour' killings each year in the UK.[17]

Like many, I find it hard to imagine how a family can collude to restore their honour through murder or driving a person to suicide when a woman refuses to go along with forced marriage.

'It's terrible, isn't it?' Dr Hannana Siddiqui from Southall Black Sisters agreed. 'It's a mindset which is really difficult to understand, unless you're extremely conservative. A lot of these families do come from very conservative societies where people still hold on to those value systems.'

Working in this area is complicated. There may be multiple perpetrators – family members and others – and multiple potential victims too. It's high risk and the safest strategy is to leave, but women may then be vulnerable and alone, with no community support. They may have problems with accessing services because of racism or cultural relativism, and problems with access to housing, health, social services, policing, everything. Attempts at reconciliation and religious arbitration are used against them.

Some women don't have 'recourse to public funds' if they haven't been in the UK long enough, so cannot go to a refuge. There are ways of getting finance to help them[18] but it takes time.

Time a woman who needs to get away fast just doesn't have.

When she ran away from home to escape a forced marriage, Bekhal Mahmod's brother was paid by her father to kill her. He did hit her over the head with a dumbbell but couldn't go through with it. Social services placed Bekhal in foster care, but then pressured her to return home to 'listen to her parents'. Her social worker even passed on a tape recording to Bekhal in which her father threatened to kill her whole family in Kurdish, which social services had not translated. This led to Bekhal returning home, although she left again later.

Bekhal's younger sister Banaz didn't. Married off to an older man in an attempt to 'reclaim some honour' because of the shame her sister had supposedly brought about by leaving, Banaz was brutally raped and murdered when she tried to leave her violent husband. Her body was found in a suitcase in a garden in Birmingham and, eventually, her father and uncle convicted of murder.

Bekhal wrote her story with Hannana Siddiqui, *No Safe Place*,[19] and together with Southall Black Sisters is campaigning for 'Banaz's Law' to prevent the use of cultural defences such as 'honour' to justify violence against women and girls. Her story is deeply shocking, not least for the failure of criminal justice who dismissed her sister, when she begged for help, as 'manipulative and melodramatic'.

She is now in a witness protection scheme.

A few years ago, I was involved in a study of homicide-suicide,[20] with a PhD student, Sandra Flynn. There were 60 cases in England and Wales between 2006 and 2008. Some 88% of perpetrators were male, commonly middle-aged white men, and 77% of victims were female. Relationship breakdown featured in many cases. However, when we looked at newspaper reporting[21] of these awful crimes, there was a fascination with extreme violence, vulnerable victims and having someone to blame. Despite what newspapers may suggest, perpetrators do *not* have to be mentally ill to commit such a crime.

Depending on the witnesses quizzed by reporters, keen to ferret out the story of the tragedy for their readers, they could be described very differently.

Compare: 'He was such a nice bloke, he'd do anything for anyone and was very helpful and he absolutely loved his children' (*The Telegraph*), with 'There was something weird about him. I knew [he] wasn't right in the head' (from the now defunct *News of the World*), both reporting on the same individual.

Lurid stories of violence against women sell newspapers.

Newspapers were vying with each other for 'exclusive stories' when nightclub hostess Ruth Ellis was charged with shooting dead her upper-class racing driver lover David Blakely outside a pub in Hampstead in 1955. The year I was born.

'It is obvious that when I shot him, I intended to kill him,' she admitted in court.[22]

But in the English legal system she faced both classism and misogyny.

Despite having endured emotional abuse and regular severe beatings from Blakely, which caused her to miscarry only three weeks before the incident, this was hardly mentioned in court. The defence psychiatrist even painted her as a jealous woman scorned when she was humiliated and rejected by her unfaithful lover. The trial was over in less than two days.

Ruth Ellis wasn't killed by a man, though *technically* she was.

By the hangman.

The last woman to be sentenced to death in the UK.

Public debate over Ruth Ellis's fate contributed to a significant change in the law which allowed reduction of the offence to manslaughter 'where the accused is suffering from a mental disorder which diminished his or her criminal responsibility'.

Barrister Helena Kennedy has said that today she would probably have been acquitted.[23]

Since then, men have continued to kill women, at the rate of two to three times a week, and still escape with a manslaughter charge for 'provocation', even because of being constantly nagged.[24]

Yes really.

Meanwhile women who have killed abusive men have been repeatedly denied justice. Provocation requires a 'temporary and sudden loss of control' and women who killed because of *cumulative* provocation, then waiting until their partner was asleep, were convicted of murder as their behaviour was seen as premeditated.

Kiranjit Ahluwalia set fire to her husband Deepak in May 1989 after suffering abuse for 10 years and was convicted of murder. Eventually this was changed to manslaughter, after an appeal and retrial on the grounds of diminished responsibility based on new psychiatric evidence of Kiranjit's long-standing depression, due to her experiences of violence and abuse.[25]

There have now been changes in how the law is interpreted, with recognition of cumulative provocation, and assessment by a psychiatrist who understands the effects of long-term abuse and violence seems essential in helping to get justice for women.[26]

However, intimate person violence is only one facet of violence against women.

Rape Culture

It is hard now to believe that rape within marriage in the UK *only* became an offence in 1991, long after I became a doctor.

I've listened to stories from many women who have felt awful shame, and stigma, after being sexually abused and raped by husbands and partners as well as those raped by acquaintances and complete strangers. Women are *twice* as likely to develop post-traumatic stress disorder than men, probably because they are more likely to experience sexual assault,[27] and they may also turn to alcohol and drugs to cope with the impact.

In England and Wales, the highest number of rapes within a 12-month period was recorded by police in the year ending September 2022: 70,633, but only 2,616 charges were brought, and conviction rates are among the lowest since records began. A total of 5 out of 6 women don't report it, because of embarrassment, belief it would be humiliating, or a belief that the police cannot help.

While rape and assault can *result* in mental health problems, those already experiencing them are particularly vulnerable to not being believed. Any history of mental ill-health *may* damage the chance of your case being successfully prosecuted.

In the UK, intrusive requests for third-party material about victims, especially mental health records, continue to be requested by the police and defence lawyers.[28]

This is entirely to discredit the testimony of vulnerable women who must be simply 'out of their minds'.

I've been told how, for a woman, after a sexual assault, the fear of a previous diagnosis of personality disorder being used to discredit her evidence and the possibility of personal therapy records being combed through by the defence can feel like another layer of boundary violation. And it is enough to make her back out of pursuing a conviction.

Although I never worked in courts, I have witnessed my own patient records requested in this way, and combed through by a psychiatrist acting for the defence to arrive at a diagnosis I had not and would never have given to my patient.

Borderline personality disorder.

That was utterly shocking.

The Home Office has once again said it will do something about this, 'when parliamentary time allows'.

Meanwhile, that diagnosis continues to be used to discredit women in court from celebrities such as Amber Heard (who was diagnosed by a psychologist in the recent court case against Johnny Depp not only as borderline but histrionic personality disorder too[29] – wasn't one label enough?) to women who alleged rape in the British military.[30]

'Everyone's Invited' has opened a discussion about how gross misogyny and sexual violence against women is becoming more normalised in society.

Even though feminists have campaigned for years to challenge victim-blaming myths about 'women asking for it', by the way they *dress* and by *drinking alcohol* when they go out together, these ideas persist in society, and courtrooms – and are even expressed by some feminist writers too, such as Louise Perry in *The Case against the Sexual Revolution*.[31] Contrary to what we've been arguing for years, she insists that rape is not just about power but about sex too.

No.

Rape is about men exercising power over women in the most degrading way possible. And enjoying it.

But only they are responsible for their behaviour.

Not their victims.

However, there has been a massive change in our culture during my lifetime. The plots of the popular romance novels of my youth where women were kidnapped, and then seduced, by powerful men whom they subsequently fell in love with (so politically incorrect now) simply don't compare with the risky activities that young women can get drawn into today online.

Reading *was* safer.

In the 1980s, Andrea Dworkin provoked a split in feminism between the 'anti-porn' and 'sex-positive' feminists of the emerging third wave of feminism who wanted to explore all aspects of sexuality, by campaigning vigorously against pornography, 'the graphical, sexually explicit subordination of women whether in pictures or in words'.[32] Even if you disagree with her views on trans women, you might have to accept now that she had a point.

Where I agree with Louise Perry is when she argues that liberal feminism, which promised us sexual 'choice' and 'freedom', has benefited men much more than women, who are told they should be *enjoying* rough sex, porn and hook-up culture even if it abhors or frightens them. Romance novels weren't a basis for healthy relationships if you took them seriously, but really, is this any better?

And those from whom women *should* be able to seek help, the police, are themselves tainted.

Freya's husband, the person who controlled and abused her, was himself a police officer. When she made a complaint to the police, she received threatening messages.

'I remember these words well, "We cannot have you bringing the force into disrepute."'

Despite a sensitive initial interview with the domestic violence officer, attempts to further her complaint were thwarted at every step. They said it wasn't rape but only 'rough sex'. There was 'nothing to answer'.

'Social services accepted his account of what had happened, he's a senior ranking police officer and very calm on the phone to everyone else.

'And I was a vindictive mother because the father was willing to help.'
She has never been able to get justice for what happened.

Not long ago, when police visited Freya during a mental health crisis,
they broke through the front door and caused damage to her home, but
then denied this, despite wearing cameras that could have been
checked.

Other women who have experienced sexual violence have told me
about the terrifying impact of a confrontational approach from the
police, when in a mental health crisis.

With the death, in London, of Sarah Everard, raped and
murdered by a serving metropolitan police officer, and the
conviction of serial rapist David Carrick, there is recognition that
the British police is not only institutionally misogynistic but also
harbours *many* offenders, some of whom clearly enjoy abusing and
controlling women. Numerous accounts can be found not only in
the 'supercomplaint'[33] submitted by the Centre for Women's
Justice, which identified multiple serious concerns about the way
in which police-perpetrated domestic violence is handled by forces,
but also on the website 'police-me-too'.[34] In my career I have heard
stories from women police officers who have themselves been
victims and given up their career as a result.

Alice Vinten,[35] who was in the Metropolitan Police for a decade,
told me how a senior colleague tried to dissuade her from believing
rape victims.

'A police officer who worked in the SAFE unit (for sexual offences)
said to me, "Oh, 90% of these complaints are just a load of bollocks. It's
just a woman's woken up and regretted her choices, or she's got too
drunk."'

Alice thinks many women in the police become institutionalised
themselves: 'I wish I'd taken more of a stand on those occasions I felt
uncomfortable.'

'Unfortunately,' said Alice of the Met, 'It's taken a woman to be
murdered by a police officer for the lid to be lifted on it.'

What Must Change?

When I asked her this question, Professor Louise Howard emphasised how much mental health services need training about IPV and sexual violence and need to make strong links with organisations in the community.

Teams must work together and support *each other* too.

This is difficult and stressful work.

It sounds obvious, but so often, as I've heard, services are fragmented and struggle. Mental health services can focus too much on the 'symptoms' of particular diagnoses women might have, without thinking about the *causes*. Community groups can provide wonderful help for women experiencing violence but many of these services have been cut in recent years. And alone they simply can't provide enough support for women's mental health. They aren't trained to.

Some feminists may believe that psychiatry has no role to play, but that isn't the message from those at the front line in the community.

What they want is *better, friendlier and more compassionate trauma-informed* mental health care.

A place of safety, where you can trust, feel understood, be listened to and *taken seriously*, is essential. And a sense that people will work *with* you, not tell you what to do.

These are the elements of *trauma-informed care* in *plain English*.

It's not rocket science. It needs real *will* to make it happen, but it could make a massive difference.

Each of us needs to ensure that we would know what we would do to help a friend, family member or colleague who is experiencing domestic violence or sexual assault:[36] how to listen, to believe what they are saying, to provide understanding and support, without blame or judgement, while helping them to find the information they may need to get help.

But *only* if that is their choice.

We live in a society in which gendered violence is normalised everywhere and promoted especially online and through social media. Meanwhile rape is being weaponised in war once more as it has been for generations.

Inequality drives violence against women and girls and violence increases inequality further, by preventing women from living in safety.

It is still diminishing our existence.

We cannot and would not want to return to life *before* the sexual revolution, but feminists have started to question how positive the changes in society really have been for women.

It's surely time for a much wider debate about that, including the impact on society of young men routinely learning about sex and relationships from pornography.

Susan escaped from her violent husband and trained and worked as a nurse. She remarried but is now divorced, retired and lives alone with her dog. She told me that therapy really helped her to put everything that had happened into perspective.

She seemed content with life.

9
• • • • • •

Locked Away

Some moments in life never leave you.

The sound of a woman screaming in apparent terror from behind locked doors, as a group of us, all young psychiatrists in training, wandered along a concrete path by a dingy building.

We weren't in a hospital, but a woman's prison and this building was the 'punishment block', known as 'Bleak House' by the inmates, as I discovered later from reading Josie O'Dwyer's story of her life in several women's prisons.[1] It was published not long after our visit to this one in 1983.

'People were terrified of Bleak House,' she wrote. 'I've seen big grown women sobbing, begging and pleading with prison officers to let them out.'

One of us, I can't remember who, asked the consultant psychiatrist who was teaching us, 'Will you be seeing her. She really doesn't sound very well.'

'Not unless they request me to,' he replied.

We used to have huge asylums where the mentally ill were contained. The hospitals have closed but we are still building more prisons – for women too.

'The needs of women in prison are being considered as an afterthought in the development of systems and policies designed for men,' said Baroness Corston in her 2007 report in England.[2] But despite her recommendations for radical change, nothing much happened.

So, who are the women who go there now?

Women in Prison

The first thing to say is that women don't offend at the same rate or in the *same way* that men do.

In 2021, thefts from shops accounted for 21% of all female prosecutions for serious crimes liable to trial by jury, compared to 8% for males[3] – only likely to rise in the current economic climate when women are being prosecuted for stealing baby food.

Only 7% of those convicted of murder are women.[4]

Less than 5% of the total prison population are women in England and Wales. In July 2022 there were 3,219 women in prison. In the USA there are 173,000[5] women in prison and, incredibly, the USA is responsible for around a third of the entire world's incarcerated women.[6] Some 10.4% of the total incarcerated population are women (including prison, youth detention and immigration), and ethnic minority and lesbian women are proportionately more likely to end up there. The state of Oklahoma *alone* imprisons more women, proportionally, than any other place in the world, and with the change in abortion law that will only increase with women being charged under these laws. Currently abortion is only allowed in Oklahoma to save the mother's life.

A young Black American woman, Tondalao Hall, went to prison there in 2005 for 30 years for failing to protect her child from abuse, when her abusive boyfriend served two years in jail, but no prison time at all.[7] (In the USA, there is a distinction between jail, for shorter terms and awaiting trial, and prison, for longer sentences.)

She was released *early* from prison, after serving 15 years.

In the UK, women are more likely to be sentenced to custody in prison, for non-violent, less serious offences than men are and are often sentenced to custody for short periods (less than 12 months). In 2019, 15% of females in custody were serving sentences of less than 12 months, compared to 6% of males.[8]

These may be only a few weeks, but during that short time a woman may be made homeless, lose her job and have her children removed, leaving her life in ruins.

Criminology, the study of crimes and criminals, focused *only* on men until the 1960s. There is such a thing as 'feminist criminology', but as a newcomer to this, I found much of it impenetrable, rather like some other academic feminist tracts. It *was* interesting to discover that some in the middle of the last century really believed that 'Women's Liberation' would lead to more women committing crime. But it didn't.[9]

Rather than trying to unpick their dense theories, it was much more interesting, for me, to follow the work of modern feminist criminologists who are listening to the *real experiences* of women in prison, including those with mental health problems (see later).

What *is* clear is how the criminal justice system is deeply misogynistic. Women *are* routinely discriminated against. If women behave 'appropriately', they have been treated better by courts, more 'chivalrously'. But if they don't conform, they are punished. Powerful stereotypes of women who violently offend persist. From the bad women, such as the late Myra Hindley,[10] the Moors Murderer in whom the tabloid press still shows so much interest, to those who are 'mad', and finally the vulnerable, sad women who seem to be victims of what has happened to them in their lives.

A real woman is much more complex than a stereotype with often shades of each in her psyche.

Female prisons have also been built for men rather than women.

Feminist clinicians working in the criminal justice system try to make changes to help the women within it, but it's difficult.

And *men* cannot be forgotten by women who are in prison, because a lot of them are in prison *because* of a man. There's often a man somewhere behind the crime such as through being exposed to domestic violence, involvement in abuse of children, supporting someone with an addiction, getting caught up in gangs or being trafficked.

A *high* proportion of women in prison also do have some kind of mental health problem: 14% with a diagnosis of psychosis, 50% a diagnosis of personality disorder, 40% hazardous drinking, and 41% for drug dependence.[11] Women in prison have higher rates of mental illness than either men in prison or women in the community, and rates of self-harm and violence are increasing. Despite their fewer numbers, women account for about 50% of all recorded acts of self-harm in prisons.[12]

I've been told how women who are undoubtedly mentally unwell at the time of their offence, *still* end up appearing in court and are then sent to prison to await trial.

Jade is one such person.

Mentally Ill and in Prison

Now in her late twenties, Jade had never broken the law in her life before she was remanded to a prison in the north of England after threatening to kill a man whom she believed had introduced a parasite into her brain. She was severely depressed, psychotic and this was a delusion. She didn't realise she was unwell and was convinced this person was trying to harm her.

Jade spent six months in the very same prison in the north of England that I visited 40 years ago. Locked alone in a cell for 18 hours a day. Away from family, and her emotional support and allowed only one phone call a day.

'I was very low in mood. I'd never self-harmed before. But for the *first time ever*, I self-harmed. I was very depressed being in prison. I never thought that I would end up there.'

Jade was adamant that it was in no way a therapeutic place, despite her being on the mental health unit. She coined a phrase that described it succinctly to me.

'Like a Band Aid on a bullet hole.'

Prison made her feel even worse than she had before.

Her fellow inmates were very disturbed and had a range of different problems from depression and post-natal psychosis to women who had tried to take their own lives and were now recovering. Others were awaiting transfer to a secure unit in a psychiatric hospital. *Amazingly*, there was access to razor blades until such point that someone harmed themselves – as she did.

'As soon as I entered the prison, I saw a psychiatrist, I can't fault that. She immediately wanted me to start on an antipsychotic. I was quite reluctant, but then I eventually agreed.' However, it didn't have much of an impact on Jade.

'There were bugs everywhere and grime on the walls. And it just reflected my mental state basically.'

There are far fewer women's prisons than those for men in the UK and there is no categorisation of prisons for those who have committed more or less serious offences.

All women are in there together.

Jade said, 'You could have someone who failed to pay a fine, living alongside a murderer. It's a pretty weird situation.'

Author Sophie Campbell, who wrote a memoir about her experience in Britain's biggest women's prison, Bronzefield,[13] was keen to show in her account of prison life that it isn't anything like the prison dramas on television, such as *Bad Girls*, with caricatured prolific offenders in and out of prison all the time. But it *can* be tough. Jade was attacked by another prisoner during her stay and bullying is common.

Personally, I'm shocked that she was in prison at all, and not sent to a secure hospital on remand. That probably reflects that I've never worked in forensic psychiatry. Other women, as Jade said, were already waiting for places.

How prison mental health care is provided varies considerably, even across the English regions, with sometimes several different providers being involved. This may work well on the ground with individuals collaborating easily, but it can also mean care is disjointed, especially when, as now, there is difficulty recruiting and staff vacancies. There is also a lack of confidential spaces to meet and talk with prisoners.[14]

Some mental health professionals working in prisons did speak to me while I was researching this chapter but were unwillingly to go on the record.

The impression I gained from these conversations was that many staff don't have the skills to sensitively manage distress and disturbance. A quiet woman could well be psychotic, but *quietly* psychotic, so seem to be 'no trouble' to staff, when they are seriously ill. However, a woman who is emotionally distressed, violent and disruptive, *will* attract more attention, but may then be punished for 'behaving badly'.

Prison is not a therapeutic environment, and it can be traumatic too.

The Impact of Trauma

Many women in prison have experienced the kind of traumas and losses that I've written about in the earlier chapters of this book.

Over and over again.

They have suffered childhood abuse, exposure to domestic violence and emotional neglect. Many have been through the care system, and many are mothers themselves too. Some are in prison for offences related to their relationships; for example, in the context of domestic violence.

Some are there for low-level crime such as shoplifting and first-time offending: things that really could be managed in a much different way, without the repercussions of bringing a woman into prison.

While they are in prison, women talk to and support each other. And in doing so they are vicariously exposed to the traumatic experiences that each other has gone through and sometimes re-traumatised. Jade, who hadn't met other women who had lived these kinds of lives until coming into women's prison, told me a little about the women she met during her prison stay:

> The first day I arrived, this other lady arrived. She was covered in bruises. She told me she had murdered her partner. She looked terrible. She'd obviously been a victim of domestic violence.
>
> Another had a scar on her neck because she killed her baby and tried to kill herself, but she survived.
>
> One was in for arson. But it was against herself. Her child had died. And after her child had died, she set fire to herself. And *that* was classed as arson.

All of this is just continuously retriggering.

For many women the trauma has been lifelong, and the criminal justice system compounds it.

Catherine's first words to me were, 'I've had quite a chequered life really.'

She told me how she was abused by her father, who was a paedophile, and by her brother too. How she witnessed domestic violence and sexual abuse as a child and later tended to react with violence herself when provoked: 'I thought that was the way that you dealt with situations.' Her jealous father prevented any show of affection from her mother: 'As much as I *loved her* I found it *really hard* to get that love from her.'

Despite the problems in her early life, Catherine always worked. There were a couple of charges for assault, but her experiences with the prison system began when, under great stress, she tried to poison a colleague and was arrested:

> On the back of her neck I saw a barcode. But every time she went past me that barcode bleeped, like at the supermarket. And with that bleep came a message. It was my father's voice telling me I had to get rid of her.
> I knew what I was doing to that girl. But I couldn't help it. I kept smelling *death* all the time.

There was no barcode on the woman's neck, and Catherine was psychotic.

I was appalled by Catherine's description of what happened to her in the police cells. She was laughed at by male officers during a strip search carried out while she was on a period, and not allowed to shower. Then she was seen by a psychiatrist.

'He said there was nothing wrong with me at all. That I was just emotionally distressed.'

However, when she appeared in court, the judge queried why she was there.

'She said, "This lady needs to be in hospital. Why is she here?" But I was sent straight to prison, where I was on remand for six months until I appeared back at Crown Court.'

Then she was sent, under the Mental Health Act, to a private secure hospital (see Chapter 10) where she spent three years.

There were some positives about her time in prison. Her day was structured. She had access to education, and the chaplain visited.

'I'm spiritual, but not religious. I found great comfort.'

She did see a psychiatrist regularly too.

> But, apart from that, it was bloody hell. You couldn't get any care. There was no compassion, no understanding. And I felt really like some sort of animal in a cage.
> I witnessed another prisoner who hung herself because they took her cigarettes off her. And there was another woman who was so mentally ill. It was just awful to hear her screaming.

She also was subjected to restraint, as she was overheard to say to someone that she might have a knife. She didn't, but she told me no one asked her face-to-face before the staff arrived in full riot gear, and I believe her:

> I was in bed. It was night-time. I heard shuffling on the wings because it echoes everywhere. I heard the shouting at my door. 'Out of bed, stand by your bed!' I was absolutely terrified. The lights went on. And then the next thing they piled in. One holding my head. Men and women holding my arms and my legs.

She was threatened with being sprayed with water if she didn't come out, while barely dressed, and was told that the video from the officers' bodycams could be used in training. Without her consent.

'I heard them say to other girls on the wing, "this is how you're behaving. Do you want to watch it and see how you look when you behave this way?" *And these are people who are mentally ill.*'

Her cell was searched, and nothing was found.

Her experience was utterly dehumanising. There was no understanding of mental illness. Everything was viewed as merely 'women behaving badly'.

That is a common theme.

Listening to Catherine, it felt as though this had all happened only yesterday. It was still so fresh in her mind and the emotion so powerful *in the present*. However, it was 15 years ago.

It seems that the stereotype of women in prison is that they *all* have borderline personality disorder or emotionally unstable personality disorder (EUPD), and they are treated accordingly – as though they are 'attention seeking', 'needy' and have made bad choices in their lives.

When women stand up for themselves, they get punished for it. They are given antipsychotic medication to manage emotional instability because that helps reduce and manage risk. But antipsychotic medication can cause problems for women's physical and reproductive health.

Prison impacts on mothers in other ways too.

Lost Motherhoods

In court the judge actually said, "what kind of mother are you?" He actually said that. He said my child being in care was his best chance of having a stable life. How could he even know that? He didn't know me. I was going to be such a good Mum. I was determined to do it right this time.[15]

The words of Mary, describing what she calls 'the inevitable destruction of my motherhood', in a book chapter that Dr Lucy Baldwin, associate professor at Durham University and a *matricentric* feminist criminologist,[16] wrote with her. Lucy describes herself as matricentric because of her belief that motherhood should have a feminism of its own where mothering emotions are respected and valued.

There are few places in need of that more than women's prisons.

Until relatively recently there was almost no research into mothers in prison, only the impact on their children. Lucy, a former social worker and probation officer, has written powerfully about how the idealised expectations of motherhood still influence the perception of mothers who break the law, and the awful impact this then has on how they feel about themselves, and their ability to mother. Understandably, they fear the judgement of professionals and the risk of losing their children, and that can stand in the way of even seeking help. For a long time, no one paid much attention to the pain that mothers in prison were going through. Through Lucy's work[17] she has enabled women's voices, such as Mary's, to be heard:

You go to court not expecting a custodial sentence. You've already taken your children to school that morning, expecting to pick them up, and then you go to prison.

People didn't *think* to ask the women how they process that. They thought, 'Oh, I wonder why women who come to prisons are much more prone to suicide and self-harm and mental health break down in the first few days and weeks in custody'.

Often, it's because they're separated from their children. And often a considerable distance away from families as there are so few women's prisons.

Some never see their children again.

I've worked, outside of prison, with women who have had their children removed. Even though I could so often understand the reasons why that was happening – their continued drug use, their choice of partners, the lives they were leading often compounded by homelessness and deprivation – it was heart-rending. Those women suffered palpable, traumatic grief as well as guilt and shame. Some have repeated pregnancies and losses – going through the same cycle over and over, because having a child was, they felt, 'the only thing I was good at'.

Much of Lucy's research focuses on trying to help a woman maintain a maternal identity and a maternal role, not least because that helps her stay in a positive frame of mind and, for example, motivates her to stay off drugs. But when they come out, women may *never* be asked by a probation officer what it feels like trying to come to terms with being a mother again in a family that has adjusted to being without her while she was in prison.

Something so central to her life.

'Maternal trauma is probably the most significant trauma in prisons. The sad thing is that it's permanent. Even when they get their children back, or if they get their children back and they're reunited with their family.'

'The mothers never lose that sense of guilt and shame.'

It seems to me that what happens to them simply confirms them as mothers who have *failed* in every way not just by offending.

Lucy said, 'I don't think I've ever had a week go by where I've had another mum say to me, that somebody said to her, "You should have thought about your kids before you came to prison."'

Becoming a mother while you are in prison is a particularly desolate experience.

Prisoners are supposed to be able to access the same level of health care inside as on the outside, but that fails to happen. The number of pregnancies and births occurring for women in prison aren't even officially recorded in England. Laura Abbott, associate professor and midwife from the University of Hertfordshire, estimates there are around 100 births and 600 pregnancies every year. She has written about the shameful *humiliation* women talk about when going to hospital appointments outside.[18]

One woman she interviewed said: 'It's really embarrassing being cuffed – sometimes they uncuff you when you get to maternity because there's other pregnant people there that are all anxious. I had to sit in reception handcuffed, and everyone that came in was just looking down at me.'

I can imagine that. I've been called to see physically ill, violent, male offenders understandably accompanied by prison guards. But heavily pregnant women?

What the women themselves say about their degrading experiences should shame our prison services. Yet it doesn't seem to. So little changes. Some have given birth in a prison cell, even alone, or without proper professional help – a registered midwife or doctor – being called, because they are 'prisoners first' and may not be listened to when they say they need it.

Only half of UK women's prisons have mother and baby units, where a woman can give birth and stay with her child for six months. It can be devastating to learn that you don't have a place in one of these and will be separated from your baby after birth. Women in Laura Abbott's research often said that it felt like their babies had been violently 'ripped' from them.[19]

It's hardly surprising then that separation from your child is a high risk for self-harm and suicide. Michelle Barnes took her life in prison five days after the birth of her baby, having spent only 48 hours with her.[20]

She had been refused a place.

Suicide is the commonest cause of death for women in prison, and women in prison are nine times more likely to die from suicide than in the general population.[21]

Still Dying on the Inside

In 2018, Linda Allan's daughter, Katie, a Glasgow University geography student who had just turned 21, was sentenced to 16 months for a first offence of dangerous driving and driving under the influence. Many thought it a surprisingly harsh term. The parents of the young man who was injured even wrote to the Sheriff to ask that she not be sent to prison. But he insisted he had no choice.

Really?

Katie told her mum about the other women and girls whom she met in Polmont Young Offenders Institution in Central Scotland:

> There are women like me that have made a mistake, that have never been involved in the criminal justice system before. They've made a wrong choice, or a mistake, and *boy*, are they paying for it. There are women who find custody safer than their home situation. And then there are women who are really *unwell*.

But Katie's family were very concerned about her wellbeing too, right from the start. She had been distraught when she discovered she had injured a boy walking down the road in the incident. A high achiever, she also had a history of anxiety and stress-related alopecia and had struggled with self-harm in her teenaged years. But she had overcome this. She was doing well. Her course said she could return after she got out. However, soon after going inside, her skin began to break down again, and despite her parent's effort, the treatment that usually worked for her simply couldn't be obtained. Then she was subjected to awful bullying by other women. Her parents had prison permission to get books sent for her, so she could continue with her studies, but were inexplicably removed.

The prison officers said she had 'too many books'.

What a ridiculous statement.

As Linda, who was a consultant mental health nurse before retiring, told me, 'It wouldn't take a genius to work out that there were signs and clues for Katie's mental health.' Her hair loss especially.

'The last time we saw her she was acutely distressed, she was crying, she was shaking, she was, you know, and she got locked up and took her own life.

'They did nothing about that.'

Linda believes that her daughter's death wasn't planned but impulsive.

'She had just had enough.'

Despite her mental state, Katie *never* received any kind of mental health assessment. On arrival, everyone at Polmont gets asked by a prison officer if they are suicidal, but if they say 'yes', they are put in a 'safer' cell without their own belongings, are subject to regular 'observations' and must even wear special clothing. It sounds more like punishment than therapeutic.

Unsurprisingly, the answer is usually no. Why would you want to say 'yes'?

It was the increase in the number of deaths of women in prison in the early 2000s, especially six vulnerable women in Styal Prison over a 13-month period that led to the Corston Review in England. It offered a radical plan for change. Dismantling the existing prison system for women, introducing small custodial units and expanding gender-specific support in a new network of women's centres in the community. Women's prisons, it hoped, could be gradually phased out.

However, according to the report by the organisation Inquest, 'Still dying on the inside', the problems and the deaths continue:[22] lack of care and effective treatment for women with mental health problems, increasingly vulnerable women coming into prison, drug use, bullying, homelessness after release, all the difficulties caused by distance from home and family, and the sheer lack of local community organisations to help women manage their lives outside prison. Some women keep returning to prison because it is the only safe place they have ever known, and closer relationships have been fostered there than on the outside.

Baroness Corston's recommendations from 2007 have not yet been implemented in England. Scotland has now closed its only large woman's prison, opened another, and also two new community custody units, hailed as 'trauma-informed', but which at the time of writing are only half full.

As Linda Allan said, 'Unless it touches your life, it's not important to people.

It's not a vote winner for politicians.'

But 'protecting the public' certainly is.

Violent Women

Violent women offenders hold a peculiar fascination. Some violent crimes committed by women are easier to understand: the killing of a partner who has been repeatedly abusive, or of a child by a severely depressed mother who sees no future for both of them. But the murders committed by Rose West and Myra Hindley of children and young women alongside their male partners are something else. Inconceivable.

Gwen Adshead is a forensic psychotherapist and co-author of the bestselling book *The Devil You Know*,[23] which tells how she helps her patients to understand their violent acts and move forward in their lives. Gwen spent most of her career working in high-security hospitals and prisons with violence perpetrators, both male and female.

Two things stood out for me about the cases Gwen described in her book. First, how powerfully our early attachments in life influence our later behaviour, and the relationship between childhood abuse, neglect, loss and violence. And second, how the people that Gwen conducted therapy with, sadly, had needed to reach the point of *being in a secure mental hospital* before they received the kind of help that they needed. Help that might have prevented such violent acts had they received it earlier in life.

Gwen thinks male and female offenders have more things in common than they have differences. About a third of imprisoned men and women are in prison for violent offences. She told me:

> Violence is a subgroup of criminality. There are a few people who are violent without any criminality. And some of those are women. But there's also a lot of women who are violent, and just like their male counterparts they have escalated from criminal rule breaking up to a violent act.
>
> Women who use forensic services are not typical of violent offenders, because they're women. So *that* makes them very unusual straight off. And the number of women who get imprisoned for violence is very, very small.
>
> Also, just like their male counterparts, women are much more likely to assault people that they're in some kind of relationship with.
>
> When it comes to trauma, the only difference between the sexes is that many of the women who commit violence have been victims of domestic violence as adults. For childhood adversity, there's almost no difference at all.

The relationship between childhood adversity and later violence is complex.

One of the things that Gwen found very challenging across her working life is the argument that women's experience of trauma is used to *explain* their violence but that the *same* argument is not used with men. These explanations for women's violent behaviour can contribute to the view that violent women do not 'own their crime', lack moral agency and responsibility, and so aren't offered potentially effective rehabilitation.[24] Gender role stereotypes are pervasive.[25]

Once again, it's crucial not to assume that 'trauma' explains everything. Some kinds of violence, such as sustained cruelty to children, pose a major challenge to feminist points of view that early trauma and/or being under the control of men is always to blame. Gwen continued:

> There are a small number of women who seem to get involved in sustained cruelty without the aid of anyone else – or else they hurt other people with a male partner in a toxic couple.

A woman may employ the defence that 'he coerced me'. But that will be difficult to sustain at the stage of rehabilitation when it becomes necessary to *own* your responsibility.

Gwen has worked with many violent women in her career. Listening to her reminded me of what I learned early on, sometimes only after making mistakes: never to make any assumptions about what had happened to the woman sitting in front of me, and not to allow my own personal convictions and prejudices to get in the way of finding out and then doing the right thing.

It's not always easy.

What Must Change?

After six months, Jade finally went back to court for trial and was sent to a low secure psychiatric unit, spending a further three and a half years there. She did eventually respond to treatment, including psychological therapy, but remains on medication.

She has been diagnosed with bipolar disorder.

Linda Allan, whose young daughter died in prison without having a mental health assessment, believes there is no need for any woman to be in prison. Her family still supports women who were in prison at the same time as Katie, and she researches and campaigns tirelessly, despite suffering intense grief. The organisation Inquest, that has supported her, say 'for the 100 women or so whose offence is so serious that they may be considered a danger to others, a network of small therapeutic secure units should be created'.[26]

That's very different from what we have now.

Many other people have written about what needs to change for women in the prison system over the last 20 years: Baroness Corston, House of Commons Committees, clinicians and academics, all with far more expertise in this field than I will ever have.

Reading through these papers and reports, what everyone agrees is the need to *keep women out of prison*. That needs investment in schemes that can help to divert women away from the criminal justice system into gender-specific treatment and support. Prison is not the right place to help women with complicated social and psychological problems. Work is ongoing to try to help staff who work in prisons to be more trauma informed[27] but while work in prison might use a trauma-informed *lens*, others are critical of the idea that a vast prison *estate* can itself ever be 'trauma-informed'.[28]

There *are* new residential women's centres planned in England and Wales,[29] where families could come to visit but they are yet to be built. The first is due to be built in Swansea.[30]

We need to support women better on release, to get them *engaged* with the services that can help them. Women's centres are crucial for this, yet most in England must repeatedly apply for short-term funding and struggle to stay open.

What is also needed is to try to help women much *earlier* along their life paths, long before they get involved in crime. That means much more work to help children and young women deal with the trauma they face in their early lives, the legacy of childhood sexual abuse, the impact of poverty, homelessness and ill-health – everything I wrote about growing up a girl and entering womanhood in a fractured world. Lucy Baldwin talks about 'missed and lost opportunities'. For many of these women, those times when something could have been done to make a difference are there to see.

But instead, nothing was done.

'We cannot,' Lucy Baldwin said, 'Just call women "complex", we *must* find the *best* ways to support them.' Each woman is an individual that needs someone fighting her corner, trying to understand and help her.

Mental health services offer too little, too late.

The world of women in prison is hidden from everyday view until, as Linda Allan told me, it happens to your family, and you see inside it. As an outsider, it seems to me that our society doesn't want to acknowledge the dark, sometimes Dickensian world of women's prisons even exist – and it judges women who have broken the law and ended up inside as weak, damaged, pathetic, failed women and useless mothers who *deserve all that they get.*

We don't want to challenge what happens because I suspect *we* stigmatise women in prison too. As women we must challenge our *own* attitudes. If we fail to do that, our politicians will continue to assume that doing something about their plight doesn't matter to us.

So, what *can* we as *individuals* do? Apart from supporting and helping anyone we know and care about who goes to prison, we should support those NGOs who *work* tirelessly with women in the criminal justice system and advocate for them[31] Write to our MPs and representatives, get involved in lobbying them and make it clear that we *do* care.

Make it our business too.

Until many more of us do, our politicians will just continue to ignore it.

10

● ● ● ● ●

Borderline

In February 1962, Marilyn Monroe checked herself into the Payne-Whitney psychiatric clinic in New York, on the advice of her psychiatrist. She had become increasingly distressed following the death of Clark Gable, her co-star in *The Misfits*, and recent divorce from the playwright Arthur Miller.

The next four days turned into a nightmare.[1]

Locked in a bare concrete cell with barred windows, no lighting, and no buzzer to summon help, she found that she had been institutionalised much as her own mother before her. When darkness fell, her screams for help, as she pounded on the heavy door, went unheeded. Eventually, after she broke a chair against a pane of glass in her bathroom, the nurses arrived.

Marilyn had never cut herself before, but she said she would do it if they did not let her out. After this incident she was watched continuously; then later carried face-down, protesting, upstairs to another – even more secure – part of the building. It felt to her like she had been imprisoned for a crime she hadn't committed.

Marilyn's glamorous life as an actress couldn't be more different from those of the women I interviewed for this book. Yet when I read the letter to psychoanalyst Dr Norman Greenson,[2] in which she described the treatment she received in hospital as 'inhumane' and completely without empathy, I couldn't believe how many resonances there were.

Borderline personality disorder wasn't a diagnosis in the middle of the twentieth century.

Marilyn's psychiatrist also thought she had a form of schizophrenia. However, according to the way we make diagnoses *today*, she would almost certainly get diagnosed with borderline personality disorder along with depression and a substance misuse problem.[3]

And, 60 years after Marilyn died, similar stories are still playing out across our health care systems.

Emma suffered from depression from the age of 17. She wrote the following words to me:

> I had been sectioned and admitted for help, yet at the same time, nursing staff would declare I was not 'really unwell', 'bed-blocking and preventing people genuinely in need from being helped', 'too young to know what depression was', 'manipulative' and simply 'needed to take responsibility'. I felt I'd reached rock bottom when I was admitted to the ward. I assumed I'd finally be understood and helped. However, the relentless chorus from staff members who seemed not to believe in my distress fed into my despair and I would run away or be driven further into self-destructive coping methods.
>
> I tried to explain my difficulties in words and was told I was 'articulate and insightful' so shouldn't be doing the destructive things I was doing. I just felt in a double bind. Articulating my distress seemed to discredit it.
>
> After a particularly difficult day when a staff nurse said, 'no one believes you, there is nothing wrong with you' I left the ward 'for a walk'. I jumped from a road bridge in a bid to end my life.

Emma survived with severe injuries that impact her today.

Women are being admitted to private 'rehabilitation' units across the country for a duration of months and even years for 'treatment'. What we know happened in the past in Victorian lunatic asylums, where patients were confined to a bare room with only a mattress on the floor, food pushed through a hatch in the door, being forbidden to see, hug, talk to family or friends because of 'difficult behaviour', and suffering assaults by staff, is *still* going on.

When they are not believed they are more likely to become depressed and harm themselves, just like Marilyn and 17-year-old Emma.

The diagnosis that has labelled them crazy, unreliable and not to be believed leading to a spiral of self-destruction is 'Borderline personality disorder'.

Becoming 'Borderline'

Borderline personality disorder is something that has been mentioned many times in this book so far.

The shocking fact is that you are at least three times more likely to be given the diagnosis if you are a woman than if you are a man.[4]

Think about that for a moment.

Men, on the other hand, who behave badly towards others on a consistent basis more commonly end up with an 'anti-social' personality disorder label, and often get into trouble with the law, which, as we have seen, is much less likely to happen to women.[5]

'Borderline' wasn't a term I heard used much in my early days as a psychiatrist. Women who were viewed as too 'difficult' to manage, too emotional, too needy, too angry, just 'too much' full stop, were, yes, *still* called 'hysterical' or perhaps 'histrionic' instead. However, gradually, influenced by American psychiatry, mental health services across the world began to use the diagnosis of 'Borderline personality disorder', which DSM-5[6] sums up as a 'pervasive pattern of instability in interpersonal relationships, self-image and affect (mood), in addition to marked impulsivity and self-injurious behaviour'. You need five out of nine different symptoms to get the diagnosis of borderline personality disorder but if you are female and self-harm you'll be lucky to get a different one.[7]

In three-quarters of cases, it's a woman who receives the diagnosis.

That *is* about the same proportion of people accused of witchcraft in Salem, New England in the seventeenth century who were women.[8] Witches were certainly difficult women who didn't fit in, not only in Salem but also across Europe over many centuries. Even in the 1980s in Manchester, being a somewhat fierce woman fond of wearing a long, flowing coat and living alone with two cats caused some of my neighbours to joke that I might be a witch (true story).

Borderline personality disorder is a strange term, sometimes simply shortened to 'BPD' (which I will use in this chapter from hereon) or replaced with the term *emotionally unstable personality disorder* (EUPD). I doubt there are any other diagnoses in psychiatry that generate such passion, heated argument and misery. It's a diagnosis that you can be given in 20 minutes or less and it will stay with you for a lifetime, forever in your records. You may not even be aware that you have been given it.

No one has told you.

Many years later a junior doctor might find a reference to it in your notes, even though you may now have a different diagnosis and are functioning well. Never mind, it's still there in print. The doctor puts it back at the top of the letter back to your General Practitioner. The label 'BPD' changes the way that mental health professionals behave towards you. It may be either a justification for locking you away 'for your own safety' or alternatively declaring you are beyond help and nothing can be done for you. Almost everyone I spoke to who had been given the diagnosis told me about the female friends from hospital, with the same diagnosis, whom they had lost to suicide along the way. Of young women known to mental health services in England and Wales who take their lives before the age of 25, a quarter are believed to have 'personality disorder' as their diagnosis and 55%

of those with this diagnosis who die by suicide are female, yet the suicide rate in the general population is three times higher in men than women, so there is a stark link between this particular diagnosis and female suicide,[9] with an average of 99 deaths per year between 2010 and 2020.[10] Most women with BPD in their notes have a history of harming themselves, sometimes seriously and repeatedly.[11]

These things happen not only because of the severe distress and trauma that women have experienced in their lives, but also the trauma they experience from the 'care' they receive and the way they are treated once they have this label.

A group called Recovery in the Bin, set up by people who refer to themselves as survivors of mental health services, developed a helpful alternative guide on how *not* to get a diagnosis of personality disorder.[12] It includes the following ironic advice:

- Try not to be female (for BPD).
- Do not argue your point of view with the professionals.
- Do not complain about anything. Ever.
- Do not at any point mention that you sometimes question who you are.
- You should know exactly who you are, be definite, unchanging about this (only people with PD ever question their identity).
- Do not change your hair colour too frequently. This will be interpreted as evidence of the above.
- If you attempt suicide, make sure you are successful, or it will be deemed 'attention seeking'.

In other words, just don't be too difficult, demanding, or different.

Some psychiatrists, acknowledge the *many* shortcomings of a diagnosis of BPD. Louis Appleby[13] has called it 'an enduring pejorative judgement rather than a clinical diagnosis' and Peter Tyrer,[14] a world expert in the topic, has pointed out how its criteria overlap with so many other diagnoses as to render it of little use. Yet many *still do* think it's a useful diagnosis, not least psychotherapists in the UK[15] and the USA[16] even though one of the great American psychiatrists said, 'the beginning of wisdom is never calling a patient borderline'.[17]

Some patients think that it can be useful too,[18] particularly to get the right kind of therapy, but others don't, and many don't get offered therapy anyway. There can be heated arguments on social media between those who have found the diagnosis helpful and those who reject it.

Whatever your stance, it is abundantly clear that a huge number of women are being diagnosed with BPD. Not only is it over-diagnosed, but it is a label that seems to have originated from prejudice again women.

Yet many of them have experienced a great deal of trauma in their lives.

Is It All about Trauma?

'At first it made sense to me . . . But then I started to become my label.'

Sue is a mental health trainer and activist with rather wonderful cats. She said that being given the BPD diagnosis (in only a 40-minute consultation) helped her to begin with when she saw the symptoms listed under 'BPD'.

Now Sue thinks it's a stigmatising term and, more importantly, she doesn't think it helps her, or others, to understand how what actually happened to her in her life that has made her so prone to such debilitating eruptions of anger and episodes of panic. However, Sue thinks people probably just prefer to call it BPD because, 'They don't really want to listen to your trauma and history anyway.' For many that includes terrible experiences in childhood, especially the sexual abuse and violence that many of those with the most serious problems have suffered.

I am reminded of Marilyn Monroe, who was not only separated from her mother when she was institutionalised, but sexually abused in childhood and became a victim of domestic violence in marriage.

Sue's mother was diagnosed with schizophrenia. 'She was angry. She'd shoplift, and the police would be round. It was a difficult, disrupted time. But,' said Sue, 'I still thought it was normal. You do.' It was a past that she struggled so hard to come to terms with.

Some mental health professionals and, increasingly, patients, prefer to use, instead of BPD, the term *complex post-traumatic stress disorder* or c-PTSD,[19] first described in 1992 by Judith Herman as a clinical syndrome following prolonged traumatic events in early life.

It recognises your symptoms are severe because you have experienced traumatic life events not just once but repeatedly over a long time.

It still isn't clear, to me, why a person now sometimes gets told they have this instead of BPD.

George, a trans man, who was assigned female at birth, socialised and largely read as a woman, was sexually, physically and emotionally abused in childhood and diagnosed with BPD as a result of eventually disclosing his history of abuse and his subsequent behaviour to his GP. George only got diagnosed with c-PTSD after asking for a change of diagnosis from their psychiatrist, who admitted he didn't know very much about it. I couldn't help thinking perhaps the psychiatrist should have found out. George found the personality disorder construct harmful, victim blaming and invalidating of his early developmental trauma. The diagnosis led to contempt from professionals, neglect and exclusion in terms of specific NHS trauma treatment. BPD, however, remained (alongside the new label) at the top of letters to George's GP and the psychiatrist refused to remove that because 'someone else made it and it couldn't be changed', which is frankly rubbish.

Diagnoses get changed all the time.

In her memoir *Motherwell*, the late Deborah Orr[20] writes about being treated for c-PTSD because of what she went through in her early life with a powerful and narcissistic mother. However, I can't help feeling you get given this less stigmatising diagnosis if you are not quite so 'badly behaved', or fortunate enough to be able to consult a sympathetic professional as Orr was.[21]

Once again, should we even be using diagnoses at all?

As I've said before, some clinical and feminist psychologists want to ditch diagnosis completely and ascribe *all* mental health problems to the impact of trauma on our lives.

I don't agree about the all-encompassing role of trauma, even if that is broadly understood to mean not only abuse, but also neglect and loss experiences too. I've met too many people who have difficult experiences in life but despite this don't see themselves as 'traumatised'.

That goes for some people given the BPD diagnosis too.

However, when focusing on treating someone with so-called BPD there is a huge risk that we fail to think about all the reasons why *this* woman is in *this* situation at *this* point in her life.

We don't consider enough how abuse, violence, marginalisation and our society's views about how women *should* behave and control their emotions all play their part, as they have for centuries from the witches of Salem to the 'hysterics' of Dr Charcot's clinic in nineteenth-century Paris and beyond.

Never mind the further trauma from the label itself, which leads to prejudice and stigma from mental health professionals and society at large.

Jay Watts, the clinical psychologist and writer who is convinced that we must get rid of the label 'borderline', agrees it's not all about trauma.

'Everyone knows people who've been in this category who haven't been traumatised.'

'If we unpick the category, we see vastly different pathways to why people might seem to struggle with their sense of self, interpersonal relations and emotions.'

She considers these different ways of mimicking what we see as BPD to consist of those who have experienced complex trauma, in addition to people with misdiagnosed neurodivergence (ADHD, autism), bipolar disorder and pre-menstrual dysphoric disorder (PMDD).

For people who are neurodivergent, it can be exhausting and draining having to mask, leading to a meltdown and behaviour that is viewed as 'difficult'. As we'll see later, autism has now been recognised as being frequently misdiagnosed in women.

But the 'symptoms' of BPD, which include feeling out of touch with reality, impulsive self-destructive behaviour and self-harm, which result in a woman being given the diagnosis, are remarkably like various ways that we try to cope with extreme emotions.

Coping with Extreme Emotions

If something truly horrible is happening to any of us, we first simply try to deny it. If I find that I have to tell myself, 'I'm fine', then I'm usually not. *Then* we try to cope by distracting ourselves, by thinking of something else much in the same way we do when facing an excruciating hour with the drill in the dentist's chair. Finally, some of us may 'dissociate', by feeling numb, detached from the world, or having an 'out of the body' experience, and even hearing voices or seeing visions. Dissociation was almost certainly at the root of many of the bizarre behaviours of those tragic 'hysterical' women exhibited by Charcot in his lecture theatre in front of his rapt male audience. We *all* use other methods of coping too. But self-harm is *more common* in women and invokes a particularly negative response from health care workers. Excessive drug and alcohol use also carry a particular stigma for women too. Taken together, when *judged* by a mental health professional to be 'exaggerated' and 'excessive' behaviours, these can easily be fitted to the stereotype of the 'crazy, impulsive, self-destructive female' who is deemed to be 'borderline'.

Catherine, George and Andrea were all given that diagnosis.

Catherine (who told me about her life in prison in the last chapter) started hearing voices from a very young age:

> I recall very clearly at the age of eight being called to the headmistress's office because for some reason, which I still can't remember why, I flushed all the PE kits down the toilet, and I don't know why I did it. And I got caught. So, I was summoned to the head teacher's office. And she terrified me. One of the things that I did quite a lot was disengage from situations. I felt myself floating above, and she used to make me

float above these things. But as she sent me back to my class, I clearly remember my father telling me off. Now he wasn't there. It was in my head, but I thought he was.

Catherine was almost certainly dissociating.

Self-harm can become a normal, even routine, way of coping with intense emotions, as young women told me earlier. George told me how he struggled to manage after giving birth to his children and used both alcohol and self-injury to contain his intense feelings. The self-injury is still seen as a major problem by others, but not by him. 'It's kept me alive,' he said, 'I haven't really had much help finding things to replace it.' Self-harm can be something that is very difficult to stop, and professionals may find it hard to understand that many may not want to because it is a way of coping with painful emotions.

Merrick Pope, a Scottish nurse has spent years working *only* with people (mostly women) who self-harm.

'Why doesn't anyone in health care want to take them seriously?' I asked.

'Because as professionals we feel helpless,' she replied. 'Unable to do something to make that person, and hence ourselves, feel better.'

They remind us of things in our own life we'd rather forget, because so many of us have been traumatised too, and we might not want to admit that. According to Merrick, self-harm is motivated by a multitude of things. It can be a way of trying to make sense of the world, to get in touch with yourself, or communicate with other people. Sometimes it's about trying to punish yourself. And for others, it seems *physical pain is better than the emotional pain.*

Alcohol is the common drug that we all use to manage our emotions, and some of us drink to oblivion to dissolve both memories and associated pain. We use drugs, obtained by prescription, handed over the garden fence, bought down the pub or off the internet to regulate our feelings too. It's more difficult than ever now to get help when it becomes a problem, yet it can be impossible to get into therapy if you are still relying on alcohol or drugs excessively to control emotions.

I've known Andrea for a long time through social media. On our Zoom call, she told me she was certain why she had become addicted to alcohol during a difficult period in her life which led to her going from a high-powered job to living on the streets in London. Growing up anxious, in a difficult family where there was domestic violence and a history of problem drinking, she discovered as a student how alcohol helped her to relax. She no longer had to control her behaviour as was expected at home and could be 'all the things I wasn't allowed to be', with the aid of a few drinks. However, traumatised further by bullying at work and having to deal with the death of two of her colleagues, she described her descent into addiction to me as truly 'like falling in love' with booze. She had finally found, she thought, the answer to staying alive. Like George with self-harm, she said 'If I hadn't drunk, I would have taken my own life', although alcohol paradoxically put her at greater risk of losing her life than ever, as suicide is much more likely when you're drunk than sober.

What did she think was different for women with alcohol problems? Well, first, she said, when she was in a rehabilitation unit just for women, she discovered that *everyone else there* had experienced sexual violence and rape. Some even thought that this was what 'normal life' really was like. Second, she felt that not only had she deserved everything that happened to her, but she was also thoroughly disgusted with herself and overwhelmed with shame. We are already judged much more harshly than men in our society for stepping out of line when we lose control.

Andrea managed to get some help, and has stopped drinking now but she said quietly, right at the end of our conversation, 'There's even a badge you can get . . . It's the label, BPD.'

This happens far more frequently to women than men.

We risk pushing women, already struggling with difficult emotions, further to the edge. What we must do is provide much better help. But how? What do they need?

Trying to Get the Right Kind of Care

Hollie, who now works as a therapist and a lived experience consultant, herself received a diagnosis of personality disorder and has spent some time as a patient in hospital. The turning point in her care was spending a couple of years in group therapy. There was a group member, a man, for whom she said everything was *always* everyone else's fault: 'He reminded me a lot of my Dad.' Hollie was gradually able to acknowledge that some of the things that were difficult in life were of her own doing, or that she certainly exacerbated them.

'And I wanted to do things differently.'

Therapeutic communities are places where people work together, both in therapy and in the simple act of living together over periods of time, to try to find new and more effective ways of coping with relationships and the wider world. In the UK, many have now closed as they were expensive to run, yet a fortune is being spent on hospital beds instead.[22]

Emma, who wrote to me about her experiences in hospital, told me:

I had been in a therapeutic community for people labelled with 'personality disorder' which I found traumatic and rigid. However, life changed for me when I went to a small residential therapeutic community that was for people 'in distress', not specifically catering for people labelled as having 'personality disorder'; I find that label irredeemable and potentially deadly.

At the second place I was believed first and foremost and then helped to understand my distress at depth. The *containment* of the therapeutic relationships built there and with other residents helped me to withstand an inner world that had become terrifying.

However, despite around three-quarters of people improving with psychological therapy,[23] a similar number get no consistent access to it.[24]

Emma went on to see a psychotherapist from the therapeutic community for years afterwards but paying out of pocket.

Sue, the mental health trainer and activist, wanted to have dialectical behavioural therapy (DBT),[25] which is recommended by the National Institute for Health and Clinical Excellence

(NICE), but couldn't find somewhere to get it, so taught herself the skills and eventually began to work for her local mental health service. Others find the DBT approach less helpful but that is what is most commonly on offer in the UK.[26] The first stage of DBT is about trying to manage your unstable emotions, and for women who already have problems around *excessively* controlling themselves – for example, those who have had an eating disorder – it can feel like 'psychological tyranny'. Then, there is nothing else to follow it. No ongoing therapy for coming to terms with what has happened to you after you have learned to control those raging outbursts and behave more appropriately. That kind of help can take a long time, and on the NHS it's simply no longer there, even though it was once.

I benefited from it myself 30 years ago.

Non-judgemental help is still available from organisations in the community. Self-Injury-Support[27] was set up as a collective by a group of women in the 1980s who could see the need for something different and better. Naomi Salisbury, their current director, told me how they still support many women long term, with no expectation that they will stop self-harming, but that over time, many do find ways to change their lives. Self-Injury-Support dates from the time when women were organising and 'doing it for themselves', and they are still going strong, but there aren't enough organisations like it.

For many, what is offered is far from non-judgemental.

Rejected by the System

Some women are refused help because they upset the mental health staff too much. Really.

'Why,' asked Naomi, 'is it okay to say this person is too complicated and I can't bear to think about what it must be like to be them, so I won't offer them anything at all?' That doesn't happen for anything else in psychiatry, but it happens all the time for women with a diagnosis of BPD.

Anya had many years of treatment for anorexia, before being given the diagnosis of BPD. As for many women I've met, failing to recover from depression, an eating disorder or even bipolar disorder can be seen as a reason to blame and discredit the patient rather than the doctor. Over the years she has felt sufficiently distressed to make deep wounds on her body, then repeatedly 'blood let' by making many more incisions. In her twenties she had to be transfused with more than 100 units of blood: 'I would go into hospital and have several units, and then I would come out and lose it again.' With the support and encouragement of a community psychiatric nurse, Anya was able to stop self-harming for five years, but a year after that help was withdrawn, and facing stresses at work, she began to cut herself again. The letter her GP received back from the consultant psychiatrist, when she tried to re-refer her to mental health services, was chilling, both rejecting and blaming. 'It would be a travesty to foster further dependency,' it ended.

The harshness of the words that have been both spoken to and written about her deeply affected me.

She said, 'In 2018, I met a psychiatrist who said to me, we can't make it too comfortable for you to come to A and E or we're enabling you.' I know how doctors become so burned out that they say things like this to patients, but that doesn't excuse it for a moment. It's this kind of awful, uncaring treatment that ultimately leads to the suicides of women we read about every month in the newspapers.

In the macho, reality of our current world, you are expected to recover in half a dozen sessions of brief therapy, pull yourself together, and go back into the world to earn a living. Anya has done most of this and holds down a job after being on out-of-work benefits for over 15 years. She is given no credit for this and is alone during relapses:

> I have partly done what the system wanted me to – I've found a full-time job. I maintain my weight so the eating disorder treatment wasn't in vain. I even pay for my own therapy. Still, I am ignored and punished. It proves that you can't even partially recover as you are judged by your past.

Now, even though she continues to need transfusions and iron therapy from time to time, Anya feels completely abandoned by mental health services that *refuse to see her*. In the UK a GP does not have power to demand that a person is seen by the NHS if that service refuses her a specialist appointment. I could hear the resigned desperation in Anya's voice as she told me, 'It feels as though services would just be happy for you to go die quietly off their radar.'

A diagnosis of EUPD or 'borderline' has even been provided at inquest as an explanation for refusing care.[28]

The police also have become involved in joint services with mental health care for so-called 'high frequency attenders', many of whom are young women with a diagnosis of BPD.

In England, these were promoted by a former police officer under the banner of 'Serenity Integrated Monitoring' or SIM.[29] These did not seek to offer therapy and care according to the NICE guidelines, but to control the behaviour of their troublesome (mostly women) patients by instructing emergency services to refuse care for those enrolled with them, and threatening legal action, including imposing 'Community Behaviour Orders', which if breached can result in imprisonment.

Deborah had been under the care of mental health services for some years, after a serious suicide attempt. She had been started on an antipsychotic drug, Aripiprazole, and during treatment began inexplicably to gamble pathologically. This had a massive impact on her life. She lost her job and her home, and repeatedly went into crisis. She was going missing from home and drinking heavily to cope with gambling: 'I was running away from my problem. I didn't know how to deal with the situation.'

Deborah was also re-diagnosed with EUPD: 'There was a marked difference in the way I was treated, once I secured that diagnosis.'

On one occasion when she tried to charge her phone in reception to tell her mother she was safe, a nurse pulled out the cord and yelled, 'Haven't you got electricity at home?'

Deborah did have regular contact with the police during her crises. They were more supportive than her mental health team, although were able to do little other than take her back to the mental health services. Eventually, she came off the medication and her gambling began to subside. However, the police asked to speak with her new care coordinator, passing on a message to let her know that there would be 'consequences for time wasting': enrolment in the local SIM service.

Deborah was considered for 'suitability' and told me, 'I felt intimidated, threatened and embarrassed. And really worried that if I was in crisis again, I wouldn't be able to ask for help.'

SIM services were told to disband in 2023 by the NHS in England[30] after a sustained campaign by users of services, 'STOPSIM',[31] who pointed out that their modus operandi was not only unethical but unlawful, unacceptable and lacking an evidence base for its claims to save money.

But women continue to be instructed, even though it's a nonsensical and dangerous misuse of legislation: 'You have the "capacity" to make bad decisions, it's your choice if you want to harm yourself. Go away.'[32]

Deborah's local mental health service also denied any liability for the problems caused by her medication, even though this was a potential side effect her team should have been aware of.

Shut Away from the World

Some women with the diagnosis of BPD are not discharged and abandoned in the community, but instead left almost indefinitely in secure 'specialist' hospitals because their local health services say they pose so much risk and concern that they can no longer be managed by them at all.

The occupational therapist Keir Harding spends much of his time now helping those sent there to get released. They are almost always women.

Keir usually gets asked for his opinion and advice by those representing a patient when their client has spent around six months in hospital for treatment of BPD. Their self-harm is more extreme than when they arrived, and they are regularly restrained. Care is prescriptive and restrictive rather than collaborative. Far from receiving 'specialist care' as promised, they frequently get the opposite from what NICE recommends.[33] Therapies may be delivered in a diluted and second-rate way by assistants and trainees who aren't fully qualified to deliver them, if offered at all. Medication *isn't* recommended but is prescribed freely, including Clozapine – a particularly heavy-duty antipsychotic drug with some nasty side effects. Hospital care isn't even recommended by NICE for BPD either.

Keir said, 'Once you get past the fancy reception areas you meet patients who are overweight, lethargic (because of all the medication they are on) and are then judged for their lethargy.'

The Payne-Whitney clinic where Marilyn Monroe was incarcerated will have had a fancy reception too. Very different from the bare walls upstairs.

Catherine, from Chapter 9, who now has diagnoses of both c-PTSD and EUPD (another term for borderline) told me how the private secure hospital she was moved to from prison also failed to live up to the promise of its glossy brochure:

> Now this leaflet made it look like a *hotel*. I remember running to the phone and ringing my husband. I'm going to this place and it's wonderful!
>
> But people probably think I'm lying when I say just how horrendous it was. How vile it was. It was worse than prison.

Catherine told me, how she had to 'comply' to get out even though she believes no real attempt was made to help her. Cognitive behaviour therapy was administered *under duress*.

'While I was there, *five fellow patients took their own lives*. Young girls. Staff were not trained appropriately, but then I thought this was the norm.'

Once you are detained within such a place, Keir Harding explained, gaslighting is common. The women he meets are constantly told that what they are feeling and experiencing isn't *really* happening, and if they complain about how they are treated, then they won't be believed because of their diagnosis.

Keir wrote to me:

> We would all react badly to being forced to live in an environment that is heavily restrictive and enforcing what NICE would describe as poor practice, yet their reaction to this is seen as evidence of their illness. As their distress and despair mounts, the more ill they are told they are.

They don't realise they are receiving poor quality care. For them, as Catherine told me, this is the new 'normal'. If their freedom is harshly limited, it is hardly surprising that they increasingly harm themselves. By comparing what they are getting to what they *should* be having and demonstrating how hospital isn't helping, arguments can be made to free them; but then there is little outside to support them. All the money goes on funding these places. Data are not even collected in England on how many women with a diagnosis of personality disorder are being moved, at a cost of about £300,000 per person each year to the NHS, into the private (for profit) treatment sector, but there are thousands. The communities they come from don't want to have to think about them, or the risks they pose, even though they are much more likely to harm themselves than other people.

Charlotte is a nurse who once worked in a female ward in one of these private 'specialist' units:

> I would say the demographic was 98% diagnosis of EUPD (emotionally unstable personality disorder – borderline).
>
> The job was very much sold as we have resources, funding, all these things that the NHS could never get their hands on. We provide a level of care that is unparalleled. Come and work for us!

Except it wasn't like that at all. It was dangerously understaffed and lacking in psychological input, with some appalling attitudes towards the patients.

When she was recruited, Charlotte was asked, 'Why do you want to do that? You must be crazy. They're just "PDs". They do it for attention.'

She wanted to work with women who had suffered trauma, but with shortages of skilled and qualified staff it was difficult to provide the care her patients needed. She also believed that the hospital held on to patients for far too long.

'They were described as *cash cows*,' Charlotte told me. 'They'd come with a funding package that was worth a hell of a lot to my own employer.'

That's horrifying. They were not seen as human beings, with families, hopes and dreams. 'Just "PDs"'. Not wanted elsewhere. As Hollie, who has her own experience of having this diagnosis and now both works as a counsellor and campaigns to improve care, put it succinctly, 'It's "Send them somewhere else. We don't want women like this here."'

But with the fortune being spent on keeping them locked away in hospital, the right services could mean that so many more could manage to live successfully in the community.

As Catherine does now.

In the twenty-first century, too many 'difficult' women are still being locked away in asylums.

This is a *national scandal*.

What Must Change?

All the women who, at some point, have received a diagnosis of BPD and have shared their stories with me for this book are wonderful, witty, warm and talented people.

As Anya said, 'I'm just seen as a "stereotype" of a difficult woman – but I have a rich interesting life too.'

All are highly sensitive to changes in their circumstances and new pressures and stresses in their lives. They *don't* all identify with childhood sexual abuse and trauma in their past, and many are more traumatised by what has happened to them within the mental health care system. Many may have been misdiagnosed, and now must live with a 'Borderline' or 'EUPD' label. They want to be listened to, believed, validated, nurtured and taken seriously as complex individuals. Many have been harmed in some way by experiences in early life and have had what psychotherapists would call insecure early life attachments which leave them open to terrible fears of being abandoned and problems in trusting others; but each still has their own hopes for a better future.[34] They all want someone to help them to contain their painful emotions, and care if they live or die.

Borderline is an insulting label we can surely manage without. I agree with feminist psychologists that it *is* inherently misogynist.[35]

As Jay Watts says, 'Cemented in the construct of borderline, I think there's a hatred, a revulsion and a deep disapproval of how we as women tend to manifest our distress, especially with self-harm, because at the end of the day, still, we're valued most as bodies.'

It certainly pathologises a way that women behave in extremis when they are powerless and traumatised. Yet people remain so keen to apply it, because it means we don't have to think of women suffering because of the lives they are forced to lead, only their diagnosis.

It's time that mental health professionals stopped using it.

If you, or someone you care about is given this diagnosis, *ask for a second opinion*. In the NHS in the UK, *that is your right.*

Possibly it's because I could identify with some of these experiences from my own life, that I always found my supposedly 'impossible' women patients such good company. We kept in touch through crises, suicide attempts and quite challenging situations (for all of us), but eventually some were able to achieve some sense of stability in their lives. Meaningful, trusting relationships that last over a long time are what really matter in providing the right kind of care.

Everyone I've interviewed said that to me, and I agree.

Beyond that I'm not convinced it really matters what kind of psychotherapy you get if it feels right, but because it helped me most, I'm biased towards psychodynamic therapy, which really does help you to explore over a long period how the problems you had in relationships in the past still influence how you behave towards other people in the present.

Most women diagnosed with BPD never get offered any appropriate psychological therapy.

I know there isn't enough funding. I have faced this fact both personally and professionally, but I have also seen and observed that this lack of funding can be an excuse not to help a 'difficult woman'.

Jay Watts told me, after speaking at a psychiatric conference in 2022 and hearing the views of doctors, she thought the concept of 'borderline' might finally disappear. It is being questioned. Views are changing. My own have. Although I rarely used the diagnosis, I have written about it in the past. I learned how to stop 'othering' difficult women, especially when I met women 'survivors' and heard about their experiences. I also learned from raw experience how I had been similarly 'othered' too at times in my life.

Unpicking exactly how women reach this point, finding better and more compassionate ways of understanding and helping them with their lives, seems essential.

Maybe it is because the cost of fostering long-term meaningful relationships between therapists and patients is considered too high, but I can't help but feel the alternative is countless women slipping through the cracks of a system that has left them standing at the edge of a cliff and telling them it is probably their fault.

Finding a way forward from this point is hard, and survival isn't guaranteed.

Emma concluded her message to me:

> I'm now completing my therapy training in the same modality that transformed my life. I've also been recently diagnosed autistic, which has made sense of many of my struggles. The mental health services kept me alive at times but with an added psychological cost – from the attitudes of staff that further entrenched my self-hatred.

Once free from prison and hospital, Catherine set about getting the therapy she had needed all along and never received.

She now works for the NHS, training mental health staff about what it's like to be one of their patients.

I do wish I'd been a fly on the wall when she came face to face with the manager who approved her hospital placement.

Tragically, Marilyn never managed to find the care that she needed, despite several therapists and years of therapy. Three days after her admission to hospital her ex-husband Joe DiMaggio helped her to get released. A few months later she died from an overdose of barbiturates.

11
• • • • •
Failed by Mental Health Care

Beautifully dressed and impeccably made up, standing with her brother, a young man in military uniform who later died in the Second World War, Barbara Robb doesn't look like a woman that would cause much anxiety to the establishment. Yet, 30 years after this photograph was taken, she was described by Secretary of State for Social Services Richard Crossman as 'a terrible danger to the government'.[1]

Robb, a bright and very determined upper-middle-class woman, who also trained as a Jungian therapist, had published a book in 1967 called *Sans Everything*.[2] This contained detailed accounts from whistleblowing staff and patients' relatives about the awful, undignified and degrading care that people were receiving in older people's and psychiatric hospitals in England.

Rather like *Ten Days in a Madhouse* by Nellie Bly,[3] who in 1887, at the behest of Joseph Pulitzer's newspaper *New York World*, feigned madness and went undercover in the Women's Lunatic Asylum on Blackwell's Island, Robb's book caused an uproar.

The government attempted to deny and dismiss her findings, and discredit her, but failed. The *Daily Mail* even sent an undercover reporter into Friern, a large psychiatric hospital in north London.

In response to all the scandalous care uncovered, the NHS started to plan better services for the mentally ill and established a proper complaints procedure.

At the asylum where I later became a consultant, it was student nurses who, after reading *Sans Everything*, raised concerns, resulting in a major inquiry, and a 'new broom' consultant psychiatrist was brought in.

Barbara Robb's book had detonated change.

Over the decades, mental health care in the UK improved due to efforts made to modernise services.

Listening to patients and those who *used* mental health services was a key part of that.

However, women are still not being sufficiently heard.

Our mental health care systems have, until recently, been mostly designed by and for men. How many have a safe place where young children can be cared for while their mother, who may have no one else to turn to, visits a clinic?

So-called 'gender neutral' services don't take the specific needs of women into account. For example, women develop schizophrenia later than men. So, by the time they become unwell, they may already be too old for 'early intervention' services, which are perfectly tailored to young men's needs rather than those of women.[4]

And although mental health care has failed many since the onset of economic austerity, women's needs continue to be neglected *in their own way*. Much of this may be due to the way the concerns of women can be so easily dismissed in *all* health care – as evidenced in research for the *Women's Health Strategy for England*.[5] And the lack of real engagement with women's mental health concerns is powerfully evident in the report of the *Women's Mental Health Taskforce for England*, published in 2008.[6]

Lacking Compassion

When women were *asked* for the Taskforce report what mattered to them in health care, respect, dignity and compassion were high on their list.

For many of the women I've spoken to, including Dina, Ty and Ellie, one or more were sadly lacking during their treatment.

Dina's experience of psychotherapy for depression, over many years, was extremely positive. Now in her mid-fifties she is an academic researcher who came to live in England, from Greece, in the 1990s. However, in 2008 she became severely depressed such that she wasn't washing or sleeping.

She sought help in the Emergency Department of a hospital:

I don't remember exactly the words ... but you felt she (the on-call psychiatrist) *really* wasn't taking this seriously. She said something like, 'Come on stop exaggerating', when I told her how desperately ill I felt. It was a woman and perhaps I was expecting some more compassion.

It isn't only younger women who are not taken seriously.

Eventually Dina was referred to the crisis team. They showed no compassion either.

'I said something about putting on weight and this woman laughed sarcastically about it. You know, I remember thinking, *who are these people?*'

The medication they had started her on, Olanzapine, causes weight gain, but that wasn't discussed even when she increased from British dress size 10 to 20. *Nor* was she warned that her periods might stop. She was never asked if she needed sanitary towels – a basic requirement.

Women are at greater risk from higher dosages of antipsychotic drugs which are more likely to build up in their body and cause serious side effects such as weight gain, which is really distressing, and periods stopping unexpectedly due to high levels of the hormone prolactin.[7]

And despite Dina's elderly mother, who was extremely worried about her and couldn't understand what was going to happen, coming to stay with her, no Greek interpreter was located to help.

Neither Dina *nor* her mother were shown any proper respect.

I could feel Dina's anger at how the sheer depth of her pain and distress had been dismissed. That she was somehow exaggerating.

She had not been heard.

She was detained in hospital for three months. She told me how acutely traumatic it was to be deprived of her liberty.

'There was no therapeutic care from most of the nurses. I was restrained a few times. I don't remember all of them, but I do remember one.'

She recalled being agitated and saying she just wanted to go home. When the oral medication she was given had no effect, they restrained her.

'It was unnecessary, I think. 20 minutes in the prone position, which is quite dangerous.'

Prone restraint *is* associated with death from asphyxia and cardiac arrest[8] as well as psychological trauma.[9]

Restless with akathisia, an awful inability to sit still caused by the medication, she paced up and down, but was described as 'intrusive' in the nursing notes, for knocking on the door of the office.

'I was grabbed like a five-year-old and pushed to go back to my room.'

There were only two members of staff she remembered by name – the occupational therapists: 'Because I felt *they* were treating me as a human being.'

When she left hospital, she was still very depressed. Her psychiatrist, sympathetic to her concerns about weight, changed her medication to Aripiprazole and she eventually recovered with the right combination of therapy and medication.

Compassion isn't the same as being empathic, which is about trying to understand how it feels to live the life of another person. Compassion requires empathy, kindness and *reaching out* to someone. Showing that you have *a desire to help them*.

This wasn't shown to Ty either.

Now in her twenties and working in theatre, Ty told me that she has since had more positive experiences of in-patient care. But as a 16-year-old after a suicide attempt and experiencing a psychotic breakdown, she was admitted to a unit where, when women were distressed and crying, members of staff shouted at them. They also 'teased' a woman who was psychotic and clearly unable to understand what was happening to her.

'They treated us like we were in a fucking bootcamp.

'They were insensitive, and not careful with people who'd had trauma.'

Ty, herself, is a survivor of abuse.

On admission she had been given a choice about who would give her an injection if needed. But despite her request for women, several male staff were allowed to restrain her. This was terrifying for her.

Restraint is something that women who have been abused find especially re-traumatising.[10]

When there was some kind of incident with the sanitary bins in the women's lavatories, they were removed and all the women had to take their used towels and tampons to another ward and hand them to male members of staff. There was even an episode when she wasn't provided with any sanitary products at all and left to bleed, with no respect for her dignity at all.

'It was just fucking degrading.'

There are no other adequate words to describe it.

Being a health or social care professional doesn't necessarily mean you get treated with any more respect either.

Ellie is a social worker.

After a chaotic period in the Emergency Department, where Ellie was seen after she had seriously self-harmed, she was finally sent to the other side of the country to a bed in a private unit which was in an all-female ward.

She told me how she was aware the ward staff thought she 'knew too much'.

'One of them was just making this patient paranoid ... just not believing what her perceptions were. And it was just making her really freak out! I just tried diffusing it a little bit, and then got into loads of trouble myself.'

Ellie has a diagnosis of 'complex post-traumatic stress disorder with associated dissociative episodes'. A male member of staff decided to discuss this with her.

Quite inappropriately.

He told me this whole story about how he watched a documentary about people who claimed to lose time and have different personalities because they had killed somebody. I said, 'I don't know where you're going with this ... ' And he was like, 'Oh, I just didn't know if you would *know* all about that.'

He seemed to think, 'How can this woman tell me something I don't understand?'

Ellie was aware her diagnosis would be challenged by the staff team:

I'd said to the consultant, try and stop the team from having a bloody debate about what's wrong with me. And just tell them to treat me like a normal person.

They're so obsessed with this 'EUPD' thing.

Do you know what I would actually *prefer*? If they could have *just* kept me in a medical hospital where they talk to you like a human, and they're not weird, and they don't keep telling you to 'take responsibility'.

I could write a Bingo Card of all the things they say now.

Ellie acknowledged not everyone would want to go to a general hospital instead. Stigma is alive and well there too. But I can understand how she feels about the constant questioning about whether she has 'Emotionally Unstable Personality Disorder', because of the implications this has had for so many women in recent decades.

This ever-present desire to diagnose women as having a personality disorder plays a key part in why neurodivergence in women has also been overlooked.

Missed and Mis-Diagnosed

It's only in recent years that we've begun to recognise that neurodivergence, where a person's brain works differently from the average or 'neurotypical' person, can go undiagnosed and untreated into adulthood. Neurodiversity isn't a *diagnosis*; it simply recognises that our brains all develop in unique ways. However, in some people this goes unrecognised, or is wrongly diagnosed as a mental health problem.

Both happen more often for girls and women.

Keira (from Chapter 5) began to make more sense of the long-standing problems she had in her life, and a sense of constant internal struggle with herself, when she was assessed as having both autism and attention deficit hyperactivity disorder (ADHD).

ADHD, which causes inattentiveness, hyperactivity and impulsiveness in childhood, may not be diagnosed in women until well into adulthood. It's more noticeable in boys who tend to be hyperactive, while girls are more likely to be inattentive. Adults with ADHD may be forgetful, lose things, restless, get easily distracted or do things impulsively.[11]

Working as a therapist with a neurodivergent patient caused Keira to question her own experiences:

> I found myself thinking, 'My life is equally as difficult, for all the same reasons.' A friend said, 'Well, you are a bit odd. You are quite intense.' And I was just like, 'Yeah, I have been told that a lot, a lot of times, and I was bullied all the way through school for being weird.'

She didn't want to take stimulant medication for ADHD after her experiences with antidepressants but has had coaching sessions, which she has found useful.

'Not therapy, but more practical discussions around making sense of your diagnosis and the things that you struggle with, and things that might make your life a bit easier on a day-to-day basis that you can do yourself or ask other people in terms of adaptations.'

'So, it does make me wonder how many other women are thinking that they're just stupid, useless at everything, or they're not like a *proper* adult, or have problems with anxiety or self-esteem or depression.'

The diagnosis of autism has also been made using tools based on how autistic boys behave and so, not surprisingly, led to the assumption it *was* much more common in boys.

Lack of knowledge among not only teachers, but also mental health professionals and psychiatrists, leads to powerful bias against the idea that a girl or woman can be autistic.[12] Girls do 'pretend to be normal' by 'masking and mirroring' and brighter girls do this better, interacting much more with others than autistic boys do. But this 'social camouflage' takes a great deal of emotional effort. Many develop other emotional difficulties and can get misdiagnosed.

This has resulted in a label of, you guessed correctly, emotionally unstable personality disorder (EUPD) or borderline personality disorder (BPD), which can then be impossible to lose.

'I think being female and having an autism spectrum disorder is a very different experience to being male. They were too busy labelling me with a personality disorder, so they missed a lot of those traits in me.'

Nicky's mental health problems began in childhood with self-harm, and then in her early teens she developed an eating disorder. Thinking back, she told me: 'I was going to be the perfect student, I was going to do my homework, and set all these schedules. Dieting just sort of went with that. I was very, very perfectionist.'

She has continued to self-harm into adulthood and has been labelled as 'manipulative and attention seeking', in mental health care.

'A lot of people ask me, "Why have you done this?"'

'I don't know.'

Nicky's brother was recognised as autistic much earlier even though they are a similar age, so I asked her what suggested she might also be autistic:

I just don't interact with people in the same way as others. And I never have done, you know, right from being a child I never did.

I can't cope with the things other people cope with. I experience them differently.

If someone touches me, I have to rub to get rid of the sensation.

Nicky described to me her 'black and white thinking', how she is 'very details obsessed', and her hypersensitivity to noise and light: all features of autism.

She was finally seen by a specialist service, which made the diagnosis when she was 30 years old after a very thorough two-day assessment. However, this was discounted by her local mental health team. She was told by a consultant psychiatrist in a ward round that she had a personality disorder and when she asked, 'What criteria are you using, he replied, "I can tell by looking at you."'

No proper assessment or a conversation even required.

Nicky hasn't had any contact with services now for the last five years: 'I'm not sure they'll tell me anything new.' She is supported by her mother and her two horses. It was lovely to hear her say, 'We just hang out, and have fun.'

But in mental health care women can come to harm in other ways too.

Therapy that Harms Women

Many people are helped by therapy, but it can also cause harm with between 3% and 10% reporting lasting negative effects.[13]

Erin Stevens is a counsellor and psychotherapist. She has worked with many women who have previously experienced harm in therapy.

'The one that always ends up being spoken about is sexual abuse. Disproportionately there are more complaints about male therapists, and there have been some high-profile cases.'

But Erin also told me about how female therapists may develop relationships beyond the boundaries of therapy, sometimes sexual, and with female clients too.

In the 2005 edition of the classic book *Women and Madness*, the veteran feminist psychologist Phyllis Chesler describes how she was criticised by the psychiatric establishment when she first wrote, in the 1970s, about sex between patient and therapist.[14]

However, in 1992 a British survey of 1,000 clinical psychologists[15] found that 3.5% of the 581 who responded admitted to sexual boundary violation, and 22.7% had treated patients who had been sexually involved with previous therapists. They cited psychiatrists, private sector psychotherapists, nurses and social workers as the most commonly involved professions.

Utterly shocking.

And we don't still *know* the *current* extent of sexual 'boundary violations' as they are called, because the research hasn't been done.

Does no one want to do it?

I know how attached you can become to a therapist. I fell deeply in love with mine, and I think he *did* save my life in the early years of seeing him. He came to mind while I listened to Erin speaking.

'Especially if a person has come into therapy, having experienced something like emotional neglect in childhood. What that person really *craves* and really needs is someone who cares for them, and is interested in them, and sees value in them.'

As did I.

This is where therapy *can* potentially cause real harm – depression, anxiety, post-traumatic symptoms and even suicide. And it's more likely to happen when there is a male therapist and female client.[16]

Erin explained how the therapist handles this idealised attachment to him is *crucial*. If he just runs away and rejects his client, that can really hurt them.

But if therapy continues, can he be trusted not to take advantage of his client's adoration? There is a risk he will move through blurring the 'boundaries of therapy' by sharing too much about his own life and problems, offering time outside sessions, his private phone number, and then even entering into a sexual relationship with the patient. Which he may even convince himself is the right thing for both.

When things go wrong badly wrong, which they do, and the relationship ends suddenly, the client can feel rejected, confused, or angry that she has been taken advantage of and abused.

She may believe she can never trust again.

The client must be able to both trust her therapist with her powerful feelings for him *and* know that he will *never* take advantage of those feelings.

He will always act in a way that is right for her.

That is the key.

And that is how it was between me and my therapist. He did maintain a boundary even though I pushed very hard on it.

But later I found out how he failed to provide that security for other women he saw after me and caused them considerable harm. It harmed me too, because the positive memory of our relationship I had held inside me became warped. Fortunately, I *was* able to talk to another therapist. Someone like Erin, who understands how to work with those who have been harmed.

But it still hurts.

Sometimes a therapist may start to believe that he is the *only* person who can help this client, or that he must 'rescue' her.

'Clients who have come into therapy with an experience of coercive control in their history, I think, are particularly vulnerable', Erin told me.

'There is a risk of the therapist losing sight of what they are supposed to be doing. Not respecting a client's autonomy, but infantilising her. In some ways becoming coercive through the assumption that they "know best".'

Harm from 'therapy' can also occur in hospital settings too.

Dani is a survivor of abuse that took place over *20 years* in a former eating disorders unit in north London, the Peter Dally Unit.

At the turn of the millennium several scandals broke about young women being sexually abused by male medical, psychological and nursing staff across the NHS and private hospitals in the UK. I heard something about these from my own patients, colleagues and the press,[17] but very little has been said officially about them within the professions. These scandals had two factors in common – vulnerable women and eating disorders.

According to the Verita enquiry,[18] to which Dani gave evidence, David Britten, the senior nurse at the Peter Dally Unit, had unprofessional contact with at least 23 women, ranging from making 'inappropriate remarks' to full sexual relationships and *even fathering several children.*

Dani first met Britten when she was treated for anorexia at the age of 19. She told me how Britten always locked the door of his office when they met.

'And then the touching started, and he would say that that was, you know, it was part of recovery.' This was supposed to be her 'therapy'.

Over time he persuaded her that he wanted to have a relationship with her. For a decade she believed this was real, completely unaware, until the first hearing she attended, that several other women had also been drawn in by him. They each told the same stories. Dani struggled to take it in.

'I was so swept away by it all. He'd completely manipulated me by that point.'

This was, once again, a specialist unit which made a lot of money by taking patients from around the country. Quite separate from the main hospital, it lacked any proper management and Britten seemed to be completely in control. He preyed on young, vulnerable and impressionable women who were a long way from home. He lied to them that he had a terminal illness to get their sympathy.

'We would do anything to please him,' said Dani, who has recovered from anorexia, had a great deal of therapy, but still has trauma symptoms: 'It literally ruined my life.'

Eventually the clinic was closed.

Britten disappeared overseas.

He was never prosecuted.

So, are mental hospitals *safe* places for women to be?

Emotional safety means feeling relatively safe with your own mind and emotions[19] and a lack of a sense of safety, both physical *and* emotional, is a theme that runs through many of the stories that women told me about their time in mental health care.

'Sexual safety' is a relatively new term, defined as 'feeling safe from any unwanted behaviour of a sexual nature and feeling safe from sexual harm'.[20]

Sexual Safety

'Sexual safety incidents' in the NHS covers everything from abusive remarks to rape, perpetrated by staff, other patients and even visitors. A recent investigation by the *British Medical Journal* and *The Guardian* newspaper found that three-quarters of the reports – 26,434 – were made in mental health trusts, and nearly 2,500 of the alleged incidents of sexual violence and misconduct were *by staff on patients*.[21] However, data collection is still inadequate.[22]

And to call it 'sexual safety' is a curious way of describing a right not to be sexually 'assaulted' isn't it?

In response, my friend the journalist Ruth F. Hunt wrote a letter to the *British Medical Journal*[23] describing her experience in a mixed psychiatric ward 15 years before.

'Even at night, the only thing separating female beds from male beds was space. This meant we had to rely on the staff to keep us safe.'

Because of her spinal cord injuries, Ruth had her own room, but not an appropriate bed. She was directed to the quiet room as the staff settled down to their meal. She fell asleep, and was woken a couple of hours later, when a new patient was pushed into the room, carrying a green blanket:

> He sat down and as we looked at each other, he asked me if I wanted the blanket. I said yes, and in one movement he lurched across the room saying he would tuck me in. I felt my body tugged, pulled, pushed. It didn't feel right. This was confirmed as his sweaty face pulled up inches away from mine. I tried to push his face away and he made a spluttering noise. At that moment the door was opened, and the light switched on.
>
> As my eyes adjusted, I saw the green blanket on the floor, followed by the sight of my pants and pyjama bottom's part-way down my legs.

A nurse helped her to dress after the assailant was taken away. Ruth concludes how she was 'deposited back in her room and in a sharp, angry, tone, told to go to bed'.

She was given a morning after pill and never asked about what happened, *despite* the impact that such an incident could have had on her mental and physical health.

She also assumed that the police weren't informed.

But being a 'mental patient' can mean you are viewed as an unreliable witness.

In England, the Care Quality Commission made *numerous* recommendations to improve 'sexual safety' in mental health units in 2018;[24] however, there is no report on progress towards achieving change. There *is* a national policy for single-sex wards, but lack of investment and reduction in the number of beds in hospitals have made this harder to achieve. I've been told how it's not easy to recruit staff to work in single-sex units because women are perceived as 'difficult'. Some women prefer to be in a mixed-sex environment[25] and trans patients have, understandably, argued to retain them.[26] However, for many women, especially those who have previously experienced male violence and trauma, which is *more likely* in women admitted to hospital, a mixed environment is potentially threatening. And for those who are vulnerable, it doesn't offer them enough protection.

Added to this, the sexual and reproductive health of women with severe mental illness, such a key dimension of their lives, still seems to regularly get overlooked.[27] They are not only more likely to have already experienced abuse and trauma but are also *more* likely than women without mental health problems to have recurrent miscarriage, abortion, sexually transmitted infections and emergency contraception and *less* likely to attend for cervical screening and smears after an abnormal result, or for contraceptive advice.[28] They are *already* multiply disadvantaged.

As Ruth's story shows, simply *telling* staff can result in you feeling in the wrong for making complaints. And several women have told me that it was a member of staff who assaulted them.

The world over, women may not be believed or are treated like they are a nuisance for complaining about being abused in mental health units.

Asha, who at the time was an 18-year-old medical student in India, told me via Zoom how she was sexually assaulted by a ward boy (a ward assistant) while an in-patient in a private mental health unit in her own country, and then sexually assaulted again by a fellow patient during another in-patient admission in a government unit.

These were the two most traumatising experiences from the multiple admissions she has had since the age of eight.

'I never raised my voice the first time but the second time I mustered up the courage to report it to multiple doctors who were in my treating team. No one even took me seriously. My complaints were dismissed.'

She became increasingly distressed. She had been admitted *because* of suicide risk:

> I remember this doctor saying that 'since you are more suicidal, we are shifting you to the high-risk ward'. Why? Was it my fault for being touched without my consent? I felt dirty and disgusted. As a child I was the one who was locked up in a psychiatric ward while my perpetrators moved freely. It was just the same.

Just like my perpetrator would pin me to the ground to get what he wanted to do to me, I was pinned to the ground and sedated with haloperidol.

She has been left with post-traumatic symptoms which have made it difficult to trust staff anywhere else.

'Basically, I was stripped of my dignity as a human being ... as a female.'

When 'Care' is No Longer Caring

Some women have told me how they experienced frankly *abusive* care.

Em,[29] now in her forties, was only 10 years old when she first went into hospital for anorexia. She spent four out of the next eight years during the 1990s as an in-patient in various units, most of them more than 200 miles from her home and almost always only with other girls.

She was terrified of contamination from food and it's now clear she had untreated obsessive-compulsive disorder underlying her eating disorder. In one place she suffered an extreme behavioural modification regime.

This disturbing account is taken (with her permission) from what she shared on social media:

I was in this CAMHS (Child and Adolescent Mental Health Service) ward twice, for a year when I was ten and again a few years later. Both times it was the same. Empty room, mattress on floor, curtains closed. Every single aspect of life: being allowed to stand, walk, talk, lighting, a blanket, a pillow was now a 'privilege'.

The most basic aspects of life were restricted and taken away and had to be 'earned' back. They could be lost again at any time. It took me nine months to earn the privilege to walk.

Being allowed to wash, brush my hair, use a toilet, were privileges too. The staff believed that 'all anorexics lie' (this was common across units).

Em's hair was used to secure a nasogastric (NG) tube in place and make it harder to remove. She said, 'The staff found this funny.' It sounds utterly humiliating. They were also unskilled at inserting NG tubes, so she suffered a perforated oesophagus, and even developed bedsores. Em is too generous in describing her care there as 'misguided' rather than deliberately cruel.

That cannot be said of her later experience at a unit of which I have heard others speak in abject fear. Here collective punishments were used.

'Waiting at the table while another child finished (in a unit that could have around 30 patients) could mean waiting there all day. It also meant children missing weekly 10-minute contact with parents on the phone and more. Unwell children encouraged to coerce another child to eat.'

Children and teenagers were force fed:

> The first technique was to restrain the child on a chair and tightly hold their nose. Eventually, to breathe you would have to open your mouth, at which point they would try to force in the food you were most frightened of. By this point the feeding had often escalated away from the meal the child had started with to double cream, butter, peanut butter.
>
> Trying to breathe and having food forced in my mouth at the same time left me feeling I was choking. Sometimes I was. No one helped me. My friends were too frightened to, and the staff would just force more food in. They were treated badly too and didn't have time for this.

Her words are very difficult for me to read without feeling enraged. Why was this allowed to go on? Why did prominent mental health professionals, who must have known what was happening at this place, not challenge it? Em is still haunted by what happened there.

And *no one* has ever been held to account for how these children and young people were treated.

It's easy to say that all this happened years ago and 'things are different now', but are they?

In the last few years there has been a constant stream of headlines in the press about the poor care provided in mental health units, in both the NHS and the private sector.

'Patients as young as 13 being force-fed while restrained',[30] echoes what Em described in her treatment.

'Police investigated 24 cases of reported rape and 18 incidents of sexual assault at a single Kent psychiatric hospital, but none led to prosecution',[31] echoes Ruth's experience, but this time allegedly involving a member of staff.

And the deaths of so many young women.[32]

Just one after another.

Jennifer's daughter Chloe was treated for anorexia in her teens and received very good care. But, when she relapsed, a punitive approach to her self-harming resulted in her being described as 'aggressive', because of being restrained and then subjected to increasingly secure and repressive environments that were emotionally unsafe.

It's a horribly familiar downward spiral.

If Chloe didn't self-harm, she would earn outside leave.

And she'd have had to wait all week for this to happen. And then there wouldn't be enough staff to take her. And that happened two weeks in succession. Then she'd react and be back to square one.

You're almost set up to fail.

Her later treatment from an adult 'specialist service', for women with a diagnosis of personality disorder, a very long distance from home and not unlike that described by Catherine in the last chapter, can only be described as *brutal*, even in comparison to the above.

Jennifer told me how, in the care planning meeting, she remembered saying to the nurse, 'When she self-injures telling her that she's disgusting, isn't helpful.'

And he replied, 'I'm just doing my job.'

None of the dozen or so people around the table questioned this appalling statement.

'A patient attacked her, and staff held her arms while the patient just beat her up. She was beaten up many, many times. Patients would restrain other patients.'

There was *never* any prolonged sense of safety.

Her family wanted her to have an assessment for autism, but this was never carried out, even though a recognised expert offered to do it *at no cost*.

Consultants came and went, and the regime changed with them – from punishment to kindness, and then back again. Chloe's arm became infected and gangrenous tissue had to be removed. Chloe also gradually lost access to all her belongings, in the same way as Em had described this to me.

Her pillow too.

'They never recognised her efforts. It was just punish, punish, punish.'

Chloe took her own life in hospital at the age of 29, hundreds of miles away from home.

Listening to her mother describe what happened to her was extremely painful. I was ashamed of what is being done in the name of 'mental health care', and the lack of action by the profession in which I trained to prevent this.

How was this allowed to happen?

What is Going Wrong?

I asked John Baker, professor of mental health nursing at the University of Leeds, about what I heard from the women I'd interviewed.

John provided expert commentary on the inhumane care in a mental health unit revealed by an undercover reporter on BBC's *Panorama* programme.[33] His response was direct and to the point.

'Nothing you said, shocks me, or surprises me, I think it just sums up where we're at.'

We made *real* progress in the past, but in the last 20 years, quality and safety has deteriorated in hospital care. There *is* good practice too, probably everywhere but, like John, I've seen how one member of staff that's toxic will corrupt the whole therapeutic environment.

It's not just about too few staff, with insufficient training, though that plays a part. Many unqualified staff have *almost no training* in mental health and can assume that very distressed women are simply 'badly behaved', that they can *just* change their behaviour, and then they are punished if they don't.

John said:

> We're now talking about 'trauma informed care' on wards where actually we *re-traumatise* patients and we wonder why they don't get any better.
>
> My sense is that the nature of inpatient environments for women are wholly unsuitable for how they present.
>
> When women are feeling unsettled, they tend to congregate together unlike men who tend to disperse and go to their room.
>
> Women might shout and scream and staff not know how to deal with their anger. So, they turn that internally and start cutting or using ligatures to self-harm. We *don't know* the best way to help them deal with that.

It amazes me that research into how to help women who are self-harming in hospital hasn't been done. But, as we've already seen, problems that are more common in women are less likely to get researched.

Instead, restraining and medicating just escalates things – winding women up rather than calmly talking them down.

In the opinion of clinical psychologist and writer Jay Watts, it's younger Black men, younger women and the queer community who are suffering the most harm from hospital care:

> As a woman, if you're in an acute ward, you're trying to get the nursing staff to have a relationship with you. Because, that's what we as women have been trained to do. It's what makes us okay, as women.
>
> But *then* we get even more of the hate and contempt and restraints.

The latest data I could obtain from the NHS England website show that during 2021–22 women were being restrained with rapid tranquillisation more than twice as often as men (women 25,110, men 11,998 episodes) and subjected to more episodes of physical restraint too.

So, what is feminism saying and doing about this?

Phyllis Chesler *did* write about 'psychiatrically institutionalised women' in *Women and Madness*.[34] The stories she tells from meeting women who had been incarcerated in asylums in the twentieth century and how they were treated by hospital staff sadly echo those I've written about here: little access to 'therapy', physical, verbal and sexual abuse.

But mainstream feminists in the last few decades, apart from Chesler, have had little contact with very marginalised women in mental hospital care. There are many who, instead, 'normalise' what women are experiencing as an 'understandable' response to trauma, but don't offer much helpful advice on what to do next.

Feminist and clinical psychologist Sam Warner has worked in special hospitals and secure units, both as a researcher and as a clinician. Despite us coming from very different places – Sam passionately argues against diagnosis in her book,[35] and I argue there *is* still a place for it – much of what I've written in the last two chapters was informed by my conversation with her.

'We still, rely on a disease understanding of how people experience mental distress. We don't understand people's backstories any better.

'Unless you make trauma the central organising principle, it will always be an add on. Because diagnosis is *still* the central organising principle.'

And it isn't difficult to see how, when so many roads seem to lead to a diagnosis of personality disorder for women, something *is not* going to go badly wrong. 'Trauma-informed' must mean much more than staff attendance at a brief course and 'we are a trauma-informed service' on the official letterhead.

Mainstream feminism still puts the blame squarely on psychiatry, even though it is only one of several different professions in mental health care.

Psychiatrists are still perceived to have more power.

Because they make the diagnoses.

There are more women psychiatrists now than at any time in the past and many of us *would* call ourselves feminists. But, in the view of Dr Gianetta Rands, who has edited a collection of essays by women psychiatrists covering many aspects of women as doctors, patients and carers in my profession,[36] 'Women psychiatrists have very much been subject to the same patriarchal systems as other women and vulnerable patients. It's often *really not* a nice place to be.'

As someone who was bullied by male managers, I agree.

The problem is that feminist psychiatrists can feel stuck between the two poles of mainstream feminism who see no role for psychiatry at all and argue (with some justification as I've described) that mental health services are harming women, and defensive institutions which will not support any real change.

Philippa Greenfield is the newly appointed presidential co-lead for women and mental health in the RCPsych. She said that challenging the re-traumatising of women in services is

> Something I'm embroiled in, in many layers. It's painful and personal.
>
> It's always seen as 'activism', too political, as opposed to something that needs to be mainstreamed.
>
> They say, 'you speak so passionately, well done! Pat on the back ... we're going to listen, but we aren't going to do anything.'
>
> It's then not just disappointing but devastating.

What Must Change?

Bringing about change in a hugely complex system like health care is way beyond one individual.

Barbara Robb didn't try to change the system in isolation. She formed an incredibly well-connected group including psychiatrists, social rights experts, journalists and leads of health professional bodies to pressure for improved care for the elderly in institutions. Her focus was on older people in psychiatric hospitals. But the impact rippled out across care in mental hospitals over the following nine years.

So much needs to change to improve mental health care for women.

Staff are insufficiently trained and there aren't enough of them. Leadership is lacking. There's utterly insufficient attention to safeguarding vulnerable women. Too few beds to make it easier to flexibly operate the single-sex wards that most women want. And the regulation of private therapy in the community, where women can be harmed, needs reviewing too.

Report after report making recommendations for changes to improve women's mental health care haven't been fully implemented.

For *anyone* you care about who is admitted to a mental health unit you need to ensure that they are provided with the proper information about their rights under the law and know how they can make a complaint.

This still doesn't always happen.

Complaints can be ignored and mishandled, especially when 'personality disorder' is mentioned. That's why ensuring they have access to skilled advocacy is key too.[37] Laws differ between countries but in England there is a right to independent advocacy if you are legally detained in hospital.

Knowing your rights is crucial.

Philippa Greenfield cites Judith Herman, who pioneered our understanding of trauma.

'She wrote about *why* there hasn't been powerful change around trauma, and women's trauma, and how you need a social and political climate which really speaks to some of these problems.'

Creating that means collaboration, not competition. Forming alliances to forge a common aim between different people, organisations and movements that might not otherwise agree.

That's what Barbara Robb did, and it requires leadership too.

Writing about Barbara Robb who tragically died in 1976, aged only 64, of cancer, Claire Hilton says that her reputation as a 'thorn in the flesh' of those in power wasn't conducive to them wanting to remember her.[38]

It sounds like she was a 'difficult woman'.

But then we are many.

12
●●●●●●

Written Off Too Soon

Margaret Atwood was 46 years old when *The Handmaid's Tale*[1] was published in 1985. It depicts women's utter powerlessness in a place called Gilead in the near future, where a patriarchal, white supremacist, totalitarian regime has overthrown the USA. Handmaids are the few, still fertile, women who are forced to give birth to children for the commanders who rule.

Since then, it regularly has been one of the 100 most banned books in US schools and libraries.[2]

In 1988, another Margaret, Mrs Thatcher, then aged 63 and the Conservative prime minister, put in place the infamous Section 23 to introduce a different kind of ban in schools on any discussion of homosexuality.

Both of these women called Margaret fuelled my feminism in the 1980s. Atwood by writing so well about women's oppression and Thatcher for her unwillingness to do anything about it when she was in power – possibly because she hated feminists.[3] Whatever your view of politics, both had achieved success in their 'middle years'.

Yet, despite being the first woman prime minister of the UK, Margaret Thatcher was interviewed (seriously) about her 'face, figure and diet' for *The Sun* newspaper in 1979.[4] Thirty years later the TV critic A.A. Gill called the academic and feminist Dame Mary Beard 'too ugly for television' simply because she was a 57-year-old woman with long grey hair.[5]

What *still* seems to matter in our society is not the quality of a woman's mind, but her appearance of aging. It's daunting that the same sense of pressure that young women told me about is still experienced when they are older. Still having to 'look good' – slim but now *youthful* rather than older than their years.

And feminist writer Victoria Smith is angry about how, in middle-age, women are demonised as 'hags',[6] not only because of their changing bodies but also their views about a changing world in which they are accused by society, and younger women, of being on the 'wrong side of history' in the gender wars.

Many women from their mid-century onwards feel more *invisible* than ever.

Yet they are still trying to find meaning in life, despite the impact on their mental and physical health of the menopause, children leaving home, retirement from work, problems in relationships, caring for others and coping with chronic ill health.

My menopause arrived with a bang, hot flushes and heavy periods before they finally stopped when I was almost 59. The *average age* is 51 years old.

The Women's Reproductive Health Survey announced in 2023 was only interested in the views of women aged 16–55.[7]

Despite being *older*, most of us have uteruses and ovaries too that still cause problems.

We still even have *sex*.

But we can no longer reproduce of course. Women's health beyond their ability to conceive doesn't feel valued at all.

That reminds me of Gilead.

So, is it surprising that older women feel written off too soon?

Menopause or Life Events?

'Whenever I tried to talk about it, I think the generic response was, "well, you're in your mid 40s, what do you expect?" Minimising what I was experiencing.

'It was like my body was changing, and that was affecting my mood. My anxiety just went through the roof.'

Chris, now in her early fifties, told me how, as she began to put on weight, she also noticed how her hair and nails felt brittle and her skin 'different'. Poor sleep also affected her capability at work, where she is still a senior manager in an organisation for young people and mental health.

> My confidence took a bit of a bashing really and I didn't quite trust my judgement. It got to the point where I was just incapable of making decisions.
>
> The GP said, 'have you had any hot flushes?' And at that point, I hadn't – but I had experienced lots of other things. So, she said, 'It's not perimenopause' and sent me on my way.

Increasingly low in mood and starting to feel hopeless, she was aware how difficult it was to know if this was related to the other things happening in her life: separation from her husband and then a significant bereavement. This can be a time of change in many ways and it's easy to put everything down to 'events'. But she'd experienced anxiety before, and she thought this was *different*.

Not long after she saw the GP, she began to have hot flushes and night sweats too.

Dr Hannah Short, a GP who specialises in both menopause and pre-menstrual disorders, says doctors can sometimes be dismissive.

'Many of the mental health symptoms that are associated with hormonal change seem to occur earlier than a lot of other traditional menopausal symptoms.'

Some 20% of women never get hot flushes, so they are not a good marker of being menopausal. (For 10–15% of us (hand up here) they never go away completely.)

'And mental health problems seem particularly to occur in women who are, I use the term, "hormone sensitive". So, those women who've got a history of PMS may also have a history of perinatal mental illness, and are more likely to notice such symptoms, even whilst their periods are still regular.'

We also know that for women with a pre-existing diagnosis of bipolar disorder the menopause may cause an increase in mood symptoms.[8] Once again, research into a particular problem faced by women is lacking.

But, as Chris said, perimenopause coincides with a potentially stressful decade in many women's lives. 'Life' is happening too, and depressed mood may be related to life events, menopause or *both*.

This can only be disentangled if we are listened to with care.

The key question seems to be, 'Has anything else changed?' If not, then Hannah says a trial of hormone replacement therapy (HRT) is always worthwhile, but psychotropic drugs, usually SSRIs, can be helpful too, sometimes in combination with hormones. There is no key symptom or sign that says, 'It *should* be HRT for this woman.' When a woman *isn't* clinically depressed, HRT should be the first choice, but for clinical depression both may be needed.[9]

This is one view of menopause and how to cope with it.

Some feminists would call it a very *biomedical* view. Davina McCall, the British TV personality, has campaigned against the shame and silence surrounding the menopause and the 'gendered ageism' that we experience. However, some feminists have criticised her for promoting HRT. In their view, this has historically been driven by a biomedical view of our ageing bodies as 'decaying and unfeminine', pushes profits for 'Big Pharma' and supports a view that it's down to individual women to purchase their neoliberal feminist, pharmacological, psychological and 'wellness' makeovers.[10]

I can understand that critique, but I think it's unduly harsh and once again feels dismissive of women's suffering. Can't we decide for ourselves and make an informed decision how we want to manage our menopause? I say this as someone *unable* to take HRT, but I do take antidepressants. We need the knowledge to be able to do that, and feminist medics such as Jen Gunter amply provide it.[11]

Chris tried sertraline, an SSRI, first, but found that it didn't address the physical symptoms. She then had HRT and the combination worked for her. But coming off the SSRI after two years was 'awful'. She stayed on the HRT but also went back to therapy.

'I think I was a bit more honest with myself about needing support and help.'

Too often, older women don't get the opportunity to talk about what is happening in their lives at what is, for many, a time of considerable change.

Rebecca is a counsellor who not only works with many older women but, at 52, is also facing many of the issues that women of her age talk to her about.

'You're caught in this weird *in between place* where you're still working. You've still got kids at home. You've got these ageing parents who you may or may not be caring for, you're getting perimenopausal or menopausal symptoms, and your body's doing all kinds of weird things.'

There are women who tell her, 'I don't know who I am if I don't have a man in my life.' The fear of getting old and being alone is huge.

The transition when children leave home can be hard.

'It's interesting talking with women who are mothers about their sense of identity, and how challenging it is when you base that around your children. Because your children are their own independent selves, and they're not part of you.'

Something many parents fail to understand.

Brought up in the USA, Rebecca came to the UK to study and has a PhD in social anthropology, but later decided to become a counsellor.

She has experienced depression too.

'I had demanding, academically orientated parents who seemed to have this expectation that I'd have a high-flying career. So, there's that pressure. Then the pressure of raising children. All this kind of stuff . . . which always left me with this feeling of never being quite good enough.'

Her parents are in their seventies now, and she is an only child. She is getting to the point of caring less about others' expectations now than she did in the past, but the sense of *guilt* is still there. Guilt that she *should* be there to look after her parents, even though they have never asked her or pressured her to.

As she says, 'That's very gendered, isn't it?'

Becoming a carer is a role that seems destined for many women, and sometimes they do, understandably, have mixed feelings.

The Carers

When we spoke on the phone in 2023, Annie was still struggling with her breathing after having Covid, requiring oxygen several hours a day. She was exhausted, 'which is just not me'.

A feminist who spent time at Greenham Common in the 1980s, she told me how she used to go down at weekends and bring logs and food and spend a couple of nights there with the women at the Peace Camp, who were protesting about nuclear missiles being placed there.

'I was always picking up on how women were treated. It was a hard battle, wasn't it?'

But Annie's biggest battle over the years has been with the awful misogyny and racism she encountered as a carer whose son is under the care of mental health services. She was accused of being an 'anxious and overambitious mother'.

'My son is mixed heritage. And with that came a hell of a lot of racism.'

She had an interesting career, originally training as a nurse, then in youth and community studies and later working for UNESCO, taking young people from warring factions across the world on expeditions as part of Mission Antarctica. However, going away for long periods became increasingly difficult as her son's severe mental illness progressed.

Widowed 11 years ago, and now 68, she said, 'There's only really me.'

She isn't allowed to know what is happening with her son's care because of data protection, so she is, understandably, very worried. It's hard, too, getting meetings with his mental health team.

'I've been doing this for 28 years ... every day there's a new problem.'

Most of Annie's friends are carers: 'If people ask us, "How are you feeling?" We just say "fine". But underneath there is serious depression. We all wish our loved ones will die before us. Does that make sense? We've *got* to try to stay alive. Because we know that when we're gone, there won't be that care there.'

Julia, who is now 74 and a retired nurse, grew up after the Second World War in a small village, within an emotionally deprived family. She was bright and was bullied at school, which disrupted her education.

'It's been a very traumatic life ... things have come in my direction that I didn't ask for. I've lived a life of being *hypervigilant*. Initially, because it was the only way to keep myself safe. It's like a ton of bricks are going to fall on my head at any minute.'

When she married at 35, she discovered, only afterwards, that her husband had bipolar disorder. Throughout her marriage she has somehow managed to cope with his severe mood swings, difficult in-laws, bringing up two children and the terminal illnesses of her parents. She is quite sure, and I believe her, that, 'he's alive because I was looking after him. When he's manic, he is very dangerous.'

He is also incontinent now, and when we spoke, was in a hospital bed.

When the community mental health team *unbelievably* discharged him, they told her, 'You're a very strong woman … you'll be okay because you're very resourceful.'

Some 59% of unpaid carers are women, and women are not only more likely to become carers than men but also provide more hours of unpaid care and more high intensity care at ages when they would expect to be in paid work.[12] Many experience distress related to their role – low energy, discouragement, loneliness and also depression.[13]

Gianetta Rands, who is an old-age psychiatrist, told me that there is evidence that the mental stress of looking after a person with dementia is much greater than looking after someone with a physical illness.

'If somebody has physical illness, they can communicate, they can tell you about pain, they can say "thank you", they can recognise their carer, they can reminisce together, have an interaction. If the person has advanced dementia, it can become very soul destroying.'

Men who become carers are *less* likely to be distressed, perhaps because they are more likely to have chosen the role than women.[14] Because care is 'feminised' and undervalued, our society once more relies on 'women's work' either in low-paid jobs, or provided 'free' within the family, and the health care system doesn't provide much support.[15]

Liz (from Chapter 8), who experienced terrible domestic violence, now cares for one of her adult sons full time at home. Diagnosed with schizophrenia, he was attacked while living in supported accommodation and is brain damaged and paralysed on one side. After he tried to take his life and she found him, she stopped work to be with him.

'He's at day centre today. Today's a good day. It's a day centre today. And I also bring up two of his children.' Twins for whom she fought hard to have custody of and care for too.

'I still find it really difficult to hold things together.'

Being a carer often means loss of another role, being a woman in the world of work.

Loss

As we age, women begin to experience sequential losses in life, of roles that have been important to us, that help to define who we are: being a mother of children at home, fit and healthy, a daughter, a partner of someone we share our life with, a friend or having a job that really matters to us – even a professional role.

Angie qualified as a doctor in 2007 and became a GP in 2012 at the age of 52. By then she had already been a youth and community worker, counsellor, psychotherapist (she helped to set up a Women's Centre) and had three children. She'd also experienced her own problems earlier in life in a deprived and dysfunctional family and had in-patient care and psychotherapy for an eating disorder in her youth.

'It was a midlife crisis ... I used to have loads of people complaining about the attitudes of doctors towards their mental health problems. I think I got to a point where I thought "I could do that."'

And she did it, brilliantly, eventually working in a deprived inner-city area as a GP and with an addiction service too.

Then her husband, also a doctor, who had fully supported her decision to change career, developed heart failure at the age of 57 and she felt she had to give up the job that she had set her heart on.

'My thoughts were that as a couple, we couldn't manage me having this.

'I gave up my career to make sure that our relationship would survive.'

It has been very difficult at times. At first, they travelled widely, and enjoyed their time together, but then he became much more unwell with three successive cardiac arrests followed by a stroke. Angie's beloved dog also died around the same time.

'I really struggled with my mental health, partly because he became very selfish and self-obsessed.

'It was like I didn't exist anymore and didn't exist in my own right.

'I didn't want to be his carer.'

There has been another important loss too, of a friend of many years:

> We had a massive falling out about a year ago. I've talked to my
> therapist a lot about what that's been like for me to lose that relation-
> ship because it was pivotal in my life.
>
> I saw my husband's health ... really shortening his life. I imagined
> my life as an older woman with my best friend, and now I know that she
> can't be that person that I need her to be anymore.
>
> And that's been quite hard.
>
> I can't tell you how I look at my life now. It isn't how I imagined it.

One-third of women over the age of 65 live alone, and women are
more likely to be divorced and widowed than men.[16] Losing
someone, a very close friend, a partner, a parent, not only triggers
normal grieving, but can, in someone with a history of depression or
other factors that make them vulnerable, also lead to its return.

When Valerie's husband died, they had been married for 36 years.

'My whole life was shattered. Because he was my rock ... I miss my
husband like a limb off my body.

'Loneliness is really, really terrible.'

Valerie first experienced severe depression in her early forties. She
is 60 now. She had a deeply traumatic childhood, with physical abuse
from her parents, and a secret she kept for many years:

> It happened to me when I was nine. And I didn't come out until I was
> 43. I was sexually abused as a child, not by a member of the family, but
> an outside person. I never told anyone because I was deeply ashamed.
>
> My husband didn't even know about it. It didn't come out until
> I tried to end my life in my forties.

Valerie recovered well, with treatment including psychological
therapy. Work has always been important to her, and one of her
happiest periods was when she was a peer support worker in mental
health, but she has suffered relapses of depression too. After the death
of her husband, compounded by stress caused by some major
structural problems with her home, she went back into hospital.

'I wasn't eating.'

Now 60, she also has problems with her physical health too.

'Grief is a thing that hits you all of a sudden. I started confining myself to the house and not going out. Not answering the phone from my friends. It's very isolating, and if you've never lived on your own, it's awful.'

As women get older, they *continue* to experience depression twice as frequently as men. Just as in younger women, losses can be the trigger. As women, we are more invested in our relationships than men and sensitive to their loss.[17] Our underlying vulnerability to depression changes too, increasing our chance of everyday events triggering it, *especially* when we become chronically ill and/or disabled. For older women, loneliness and depression are linked[18] and if, like Valerie, you've had episodes of depression previously, this increases the likelihood of it returning.

In the UK, the peak suicide rate for women is currently between ages 50 and 54[19] and in the USA between 45 and 64[20] but we still don't really understand enough about why, even though it is a time of considerable change. For women aged 45–54 without a degree education in the USA, the changes over the last 30 years are stark. In 1992 they were more likely to die of heart disease than die from drugs, alcohol or social isolation. Now they are 30% more likely to die from what have been called 'deaths of despair'.[21]

Carolyn Chew-Graham, my GP friend, told me how older people are less likely to come forward and ask for help with depression, but it *is* easier to raise with women than men.

Nevertheless, older people in general are much less likely to get access to psychological therapies, because there is still a belief among many that they don't benefit, when they do! And women, especially older women, are more likely to be treated with electroconvulsive therapy (ECT) than men.

Does this mean that women are being violently punished with ECT as some feminists have claimed? Or is it more complicated than that?

ECT: Dangerous Punishment . . . or Lifesaving?

Reading accounts of ECT from the past, it's not difficult to see how veteran feminist and 'anti-psychiatrist', the late Bonnie Burstow, concluded that ECT should be banned because she believed it to be a tool of punishment and control which constituted violence against women.[22]

It is one of the last remaining practices of the 'old' days of psychiatry, and popular images of it are still anchored to the horrific scene in *One Flew Over the Cuckoo's Nest* when it is given with neither general anaesthesia nor a muscle relaxant, as indeed it once was.[23]

So, I *can* understand the fear.

I *also* don't doubt whatsoever that people *have* been harmed by ECT in the past when it wasn't delivered with as much care as it is now[24] and may still be where it is not given safely. My own experiences of some patients receiving it in the 1980s, when I wasn't always convinced it was the right treatment, would have left me sceptical too (see Chapter 5), had it not been for one thing.

I saw it work extremely effectively in people for whom nothing else seemed to help.

Tania Gergel estimates she has been given ECT more than 200 times over the last 30 years. Now 51, she has bipolar disorder that doesn't respond to *anything* other than ECT. When she is unwell, she becomes psychotic, has racing thoughts going so fast that it feels like her brain will explode and her 'urge to self-destruct is absolute'.

'It's like a wall comes down between myself and reality.'

Medication does nothing.

ECT is usually given twice a week over 3–5 weeks. The first time she had it she said that, 'After about the fifth or the sixth one, I suddenly woke up. And it was as if that wall had just gone . . . I was back in the world, and I no longer was experiencing psychosis. I wasn't suicidal anymore.'

Between her episodes of illness, she has had a very successful career as an academic. But there have been side effects. Gaps in her 'autobiographical memory', the memories of her own life, from both just before treatment and during it. Some of these gaps have been permanent. But she can still form new memories, and there has been no impact on her ability to reason and think. She *is* critical of psychiatrists who try to minimise the side effects. They are *real*, and a decision about ECT always needs the costs and benefits for that person weighing up.[25] However, Tania is also critical of anti-ECT polemic which suggests lack of effectiveness and inaccurate or exaggerated risks.

'The attack against ECT is a kind of generalised psychiatry *conspiracy theory*. And part of conspiracy theory is the idea that you're keeping silent about stuff.'

That seems to be what others who have taken up Bonnie Burstow's campaign to ban ECT, citing how it is given disproportionately to women, seem to claim.[26] However, it's worth noting that some of those who seek to ban it do not acknowledge that 'mental illness', never mind the severe kind of illness Tania has experienced, exists.

There *is* evidence that ECT works[27] and oversight of it in the UK has improved vastly over the last 40 years. Women *do* receive two-thirds of all ECT treatments, because depression is twice as common in women as in men. The average age for treatment with ECT is 61 years because older women do receive it more frequently than younger women. Older people can become dangerously unwell with depression and stop eating and drinking. NICE says that ECT should be used if the person prefers to have it based on past experience, if a rapid response is needed and if *other treatments have failed.*[28] If they are unable to give informed consent, then there are strict guidelines under mental health legislation to be followed before it can be given in the UK.[29]

If ECT were banned, what would happen to women like Tania for whom it's the only thing that works? What would happen to those older women with severe depression who believe that they cannot eat or drink because their insides have rotted away? To the suicidal women stuck in severe depression for months or years and *not* helped by any other treatment? To StrongestSmile in Chapter 4 who believes that without it she would also not be here?

ECT can be lifesaving.

We risk writing off many women too soon by *not* using it.

However, as we age, we are aware of our increasing physical and mental frailty.

Will Our Health Problems Be Taken Seriously?

Older women worry about what will happen to our bodies and minds as we age – how we will cope and be treated by health care providers.

Jude, nearly 60, who has done *many* different things in her life, is still working, as consultant mediator and coach in the English NHS. She broke three bones in her foot recently while on holiday:

> They were saying, 'Oooh, you're 60, you need a dexa scan' (for bone density). The attitude of some of the staff ... because I was approaching 60, they thought I was *old*. I was frail! 'How many falls have you had they asked?' Nobody asked me how I had fallen or where or when? The fact that I was on a long-distance walking trip and fell down a ravine didn't get a mention! So, there's a *change* isn't there, in other people's assumptions.

They begin to view us differently.

Some health problems that older women experience aren't taken as seriously as they should be by doctors. Other problems experienced by women don't receive as much research investment. They aren't taken as seriously by our society.

Let's consider two very different problems: fibromyalgia and dementia.

Julia, the 74-year-old retired nurse who has spent many years caring for her husband, was diagnosed with an inherited chronic kidney disease in her forties which caused episodes of severe pain and she had to do home dialysis for some time before having a kidney transplant. She has now been diagnosed with heart disease too.

Somehow, she has managed to keep going.

And, as if all this wasn't enough, five years ago she was also diagnosed with fibromyalgia too.

Fibromyalgia is more common in women than in men and most often diagnosed in middle age. It causes pain and fatigue as well as mood problems.[30] It's particularly problematic for women because for many years it was considered purely 'psychological'. We don't fully understand what causes it, and it can still be difficult to get help.

Freida, from Chapter 7, and who is now 65, also has fibromyalgia. She told me how when she first complained of pains in her arms, 'my doctors first thought it was "all in my head". When my fibromyalgia pain gets *real* bad, sometimes it will trigger my anxiety and then I start having headaches.'

Freida dates the onset of her problems from when she had an accident and injured her back.

'It takes some trauma to trigger it.'

That can be physical, like an infection, or emotional – a life event. Or maybe there will be nothing at all that can be identified. But like many women I have met over decades with persistent physical symptoms, Freida has lived a difficult life. Not only subject to repeated physical trauma but sexual violence and racial discrimination.

Pain may be 'embodied', in that it becomes a woman's way of experiencing a world that is full of pain. How we cope with that pain, however, can become controversial. Trying to suppress it, particularly with medication, can mean accusations of buying into the 'neoliberal' idea that we must live happy, pain-free lives. When I hear this, I wonder if those who say it have experienced real suffering. I know women who have severe chronic pain and are offered psychological therapies to help them 'manage' it, which do nothing for them. They are *not* assuming a victim role. The struggle to find the best way of living with pain can be a long journey.[31]

Julia Hose, a psychiatrist who specialises in helping people with persistent physical symptoms told me, 'When you are trying to get a diagnosis, everything is made worse by the attitudes of health care professionals, particularly if you are a woman and if you're a woman of colour. Doctors can be incredibly dismissive.'

The symptoms are *real* and not being faked.

'*All* symptoms have a psychological component,' even when the cause *is* quite clear.

'But there's still a lot of blaming. This is your fault.'

This is your problem.

'You become a "difficult woman" if you've been traumatised, or if you've been treated badly by the health care system repeatedly. No matter what you say, it will be viewed within the framework of you're being difficult, or you're awkward, or you just want money, you're drug seeking, or you're "dependent". I hate that word.'

It is a term of abuse.

Being told it is 'your problem' by the medical profession and to not 'invest in victimhood' by some feminists[32] just compounds the suffering.

No wonder some women feel written off.

Dementia is a very different problem. We know what causes it. It is a disease of the brain that affects our memory, ability to think and our behaviour.

There are several different types of dementia,[33] but Alzheimer's disease is the most common, and there are *twice* as many women as men over 65 years old who suffer it.

I was taught this was because women live longer, but we don't know if that is really true.

A recent study suggests that genetic factors may contribute to the high rate in women.[34] We know that early menopause can also increase the risk. But research into dementia has received much less research funding[35] than other diseases such as cancer and cardiovascular disease, despite the massive impact it has on society – and on *women* in particular.

Not only are women the majority of those who are carers for people with dementia, but they are also the majority of those who will live out their days in care homes and hospital suffering from dementia.

Dementia is the leading cause of death for women in England and Wales.[36]

Do we not matter as much?

Margaret Thatcher, the former prime minister, suffered from dementia before her death. In 2008 her daughter revealed that her memory had been declining for several years.[37] She would ask the same question repeatedly, unaware that it had been answered. She forgot that her husband had died. Her short-term memory had failed, but she could still remember the more distant past. That she had an intellectually demanding life might have helped to delay the onset of dementia.

She finally died from a stroke in 2013, aged 87.

Gianetta Rands, the old-age psychiatrist, told me how when confused and disinhibited by dementia, some women in hospital begin to talk about their experiences from the past, sometimes revealing long-kept secrets about abuse, terminations and secret pregnancies. Talking about things that had happened to them as young women growing up in the world of their time, things that would never have crossed the mind of their family members.

Many of the women with dementia she cared for in hospital had been abused earlier in their life – mostly sexually.

'It was as if the ones who had been abused in childhood, didn't have the emotional and psychological resources to find a way out of hospital or not get into hospital, or to cope with the burdens of getting older.'

Even in old age and suffering from dementia, the things that have happened to us in our distant past are still held within us.

Many older women are *survivors* of the multiple struggles I've described in this book.

Survivors

In *Not Dead Yet*[38] (such a marvellous title), Renate Klein and Susan Hawthorne have collected contributions – memoir, history, poetry and snapshots of present lives – from many pioneering second-wave feminists, who are all over 70 years old. They still have revolutionary zest. They are *angry* about how 'history is being rewritten'. However, many woman of a similar age would also find much to disagree with them about too. They represent a *particular* view of what feminism was and is. They also don't say much about mental health in old age.

Feminism really hasn't.

There are some parallels between the women of *Not Dead Yet* and the lives of the women who have spoken to me, particularly on the thorny questions of the gender wars, and whether younger women appreciate the battle that second-wave feminists fought during the 1960s to 1980s. However, *our* conversations were not only about the past but also about surviving in the present and finding ways to keep going in the future in the world as it is *now*.

They are not going to be 'written off', either.

Chris, who struggled with her menopause, is passionate about women's health in the workplace and outside it. We talked about our shared belief that women need services to take into consideration the demands they face in their lives: childcare and other caring responsibilities; practical problems such as trying to reach a distant hospital on public transport with small children. She also told me: 'I've spoken to my boss about whether we should have a menopause policy. And she said, Yeah, great. Go ahead. Write one!'

Valerie, who was bereaved, was very clear about needing a purpose in her life after retirement. She does voluntary work for the local foodbank, befriending, and helped to design a course with the university to train approved mental health practitioners who have responsibilities under mental health law. On the course, she discusses candidly her own personal experiences of being detained in hospital.

Angie, who gave up her career as a doctor when her husband fell ill, rediscovered her love of painting. She goes away for holidays with girlfriends and for massages, and she enjoys being with her family too. There's a grandchild on the way.

'I've found other ways to be me.' But people still ask, 'Can you just have a look at this mole.'

Rediscovering creativity matters. Rebecca, who is still working as a counsellor, also does writing for wellbeing workshops and is a published fiction writer.

'You're taking the stuff out of your head, and you're putting it there, on the page, where you can look at it a bit more objectively.'

There are parallels between therapy and writing, and she thinks the latter has probably helped the most.

Julia, freed from being a carer of her husband at the time we spoke, has learned to play the drums. She told me how, after her kidney transplant, she sensed she had 'come alive' again and she wants to discover who her 'inner child' really is.

For some, the struggle to survive is harder, and the future even more uncertain.

This is true for both Fiona and Nessa.

Fiona, now 55, advises on research into older people who self-harm and is concerned that there is nothing targeted at helping older people. She began to cut herself at the age of 14 but hasn't self-harmed for a long time though it could happen again if she is under stress.

'I use it as a form of coping.'

'As I get older, how many people will then be involved in my care? I might not be able to use it for stress relief.'

An Anglican priest, Fiona was formerly a social worker. Both challenging roles for someone who was adopted by an older couple who chose her from a group photograph, when her single parent birth mother had, she discovered later, tried to keep them together for six months.

Adoption in the mid 1960s was, for her, an awful experience.

'My mother had definite views. Boys could do no wrong and my role in life was to become the housewife, the breeder.'

She was bright. The boy, her adoptive brother, was jealous and abusive.

At 14 she went into care, and, by then 'out of control', neither went to school nor returned home. Leaving care at 18 she used her grant not for a bedsit as it was intended, but a sailing qualification, travelling the world by boat for three years and discovering she was a 'nice, compassionate, loyal' person after all. Then, after re-accessing education and 10 years as a social worker, began training as a priest.

'I wanted to be a better social worker. I think I was – but it was at such a cost to me, not only with the whole thing about vicarious trauma, but also because of my background.'

'How have I managed to survive until now?'

Fiona was initially diagnosed as having recurrent depression. Then re-diagnosed with EUPD.

'I was irritable. I was a social worker, of course, I was!'

Her GP saw her when she was clearly hypomanic. She almost certainly focused her hypomanic energy into work. But the mental health team said *they* hadn't seen her when she was overactive and full of energy.

In 2016 she saw a respected psychiatrist privately who diagnosed her with bipolar disorder. She now remains well if she stays on medication, but the local mental health service doesn't accept her re-diagnosis and have discharged her. This is despite an episode when, having stopped her medication, she became very severely depressed and was detained in hospital in Scotland, where she had travelled intending to take her life.

I fully appreciate Fiona's fears for the future.

She now has multiple physical health problems too. Her husband is her major support and she is getting older.

'My concerns are that he's going to become unwell and I'm going to have to care for him . . .

'In the middle of the night, I wake up thinking what would I do if . . . ?'

I understand that too well.

Nessa's is the final story I will tell in this book.

It greatly affected me and has lingered in my mind.

'I entered the psychiatric system in 1993. I'd just graduated,' Nessa told me, 'With zero understanding and zero self-awareness.

'I was given various diagnoses.

'Then borderline personality disorder stuck for well, 27 years.'

Nessa's problems also began in her traumatic childhood. She had anorexia 'quite badly'. She took overdoses and self-harmed. She has twice been in intensive care.

'I exhibited challenging behaviour. I was "untreatable." I had no idea why I was like that apart from that I was a bad person. Nobody tried to point out to me that there may be reasons for my behaviour.

'I was desperate to self-destruct.'

Her weight has plummeted dangerously at times. At one point in the 1990s she was force-fed. She says she thought it was what she deserved. She was given ECT and it didn't help. All of this simply reinforced her original trauma. She was in and out of hospital for a decade.

Then she spent some time in a therapeutic community. It seemed to help her become more conscious of what she had been through. After that, she did 'fairly well' for a period, caring for her grandparents and training as a nurse. But she was awfully aware of wanting to be cared for, rather than doing the caring, and dropped out after two years.

Her first specialist eating disorder admission only happened when she was 43.

'I talked about a few things which acted as a catalyst to things like police investigations, stuff in my past, and so it all kind of snowballed, but I wasn't getting any help.'

'It's been a system that doesn't understand, with a person that doesn't understand. I've survived just by sheer dogged determination.'

She now has a diagnosis of complex post-traumatic stress disorder and dissociative identity disorder. Two years of private counselling helped her to see herself in a 'better light'. However, having been at least 'held' by mental health services, who provided a necessary safety net for 27 years, she was discharged in 2019 without warning when still very vulnerable and on multiple medications. She considered suicide but said she would never leave her dog.

At 52, Nessa has survived and fought for her voice to be heard but still doesn't feel she is listened to or taken seriously.

'What a scary, lonely fight it's been ... I want to use my whole existence as a legacy. *I just want some good to come out of it.*'

I've heard many stories of other women at different stages on the same journey that Fiona and Nessa have been travelling for 50 years. They have survived, but the system has deserted them.

I worry about how they will fare as they grow older and fear the repetition of this terrible cycle of neglect.

What Must Change?

A strategy for women's health[39] must ensure that it isn't too focused on reproduction and remembers the mental health and physical health of older women, and especially how women's *pain* is so easily dismissed at any age.

Changing a world which is not only sexist, but also ageist and discriminatory in a myriad of other ways is a massive enterprise. But simply providing more positive images of older women in the media, active and enjoying life rather than curled up in a chair in a nursing home, written off by the world, might be a small beginning. The Centre for Aging Better[40] has collected a massive library of pictures of people, over the age of 50 who are still engaged in life, 'invisible' older women at work.

We are here and we want to be seen.

Caring isn't just a problem for women, it's a human problem.[41]

The plight of women who are carers, and have to give up work, could and should be improved. Much more effort needs to put into supporting carers to be able to stay in work and creating carer-friendly workplaces.[42] From 2024, carers are going to be entitled to one week's unpaid leave in the UK. Not only should it be *paid*, but also policies are considerably more generous and flexible in some other countries.[43]

Longer term, perhaps one day there will be a solution to the funding of social care in society such that it doesn't rely on the unpaid and/or outrageously low-paid work of women (but I'm not holding my breath).

For feminism, the young women of today will be the older women of tomorrow, and maintaining connection between younger and older women seems important.

Some older feminists find that divisions over gender politics get in the way. Susan Faludi has even suggested that women are facing a war on two fronts, not only in a battle of the sexes but also in a battle of the ages,[44] as young women reject the values of their mothers. Yet isn't that something that my generation did too? That all generations do? To enforce one's values on another seems like just another form of patriarchy to me (or matriarchy?).

I know that's hard, but we must not allow our disagreements to get in the way of supporting younger women to live in this world, and allowing them to get to know us better, while making their *own* choices. Because there are things older women can both share with, and learn from, younger ones.

Together we can perhaps begin to work out what 'feminist old age' really looks like,[45] and how it *will* change for future generations. But there are several examples above from my interviewees. What women have told me is that gender stereotypes matter less as you age, or to put it succinctly, as Chris said to me about her peri-menopausal life, 'I'm not giving so much of a shit about what other people think.'

For ourselves, and those we love, there are things we can do to reduce our risk of getting dementia.[46] 'Keep moving,' as a GP said to me recently. It's never too late to stop smoking. Try to eat healthily and cut down on alcohol. Hopefully, these will help us live longer too (although I admit it may just seem like it to some).

But we can try to take control of our health and *stay connected* with the world. 'I don't want to be stuck at home,' Angie the former GP told me. 'I want to be part of what's going on!'

And before it's too late for them to easily learn, help older women you know to access the internet so they can stay engaged.

It may be lifesaving.

In 2019, a 79-year-old Margaret Attwood jointly won the Booker Prize (with Bernadine Evaristo) for *The Testaments*. Attwood was oldest woman and Evaristo, at 60, the first Black woman to win.

The Testaments[47] was the long-awaited sequel to The Handmaid's Tale.

Together they tell a story of *survival*: of discovering ways to keep going against the odds and finding hope in the depths of despair.

Conclusion

Scotland 2024

A great deal has happened since that evening in Manchester when we debated whether 'Men are the losers now' in front of an audience for 'Woman's Week'.

On a personal level, I now live on a Scottish island. Like many older women, I went grey during the pandemic, *not* from stress, although that was considerable, but lack of access to a hairdresser. I have finally given up trying to look younger than my years.

But these are the minor concerns of a privileged northern European white woman.

Far, far more serious things have been going on in the world.

In Afghanistan, women are now prevented from accessing *education* beyond primary school. Following the overturning of *Roe v. Wade*, in the USA the state of Texas is planning to stop pregnant women travelling across the state border to end 'abortion trafficking'.[1]

Across the world, the pandemic *did* demonstrate that the gains feminism made in gender equality had shaky foundations when it became clear that women carried the burden of the impact of Covid-19 on families.

Misogyny flourishes in the world that gave us Trump and may return that gift again.

All of these will have a significant impact on women's mental health. Things *are* getting worse. Especially for young women trying to navigate growing up in a world where young people (especially men) learn about sexual behaviour and (lack of) consent from pornography.

We *must* speak out about it.

But when women complain about our lives are told we are 'out of our minds'.

I reiterate, this can mean three different things. Written off as merely 'crazy' anyway and wasting time. Simply driven to that point by the ways in which we are treated. Or our reaction on discovering that our mental health problems are apparently *less important*.

Let's take them one at a time.

First, we are NOT crazy when we need to talk about the kinds of pain, suffering, abuse, violence and fear that women have spoken about here. These are not *our fault*. We should not be ignored, blamed or viewed as 'wasting time'.

We have a right to support and care as equal human beings.

Second, women are oppressed in a multitude of different ways even within our 'liberal' societies.

For many, especially those who suffer abuse early in their lives then struggle through economic hardship and violence as adults, it's not surprising at all that they suffer with their mental health. But they still often don't get taken seriously when they ask for help. *They* become seen as the problem, rather than the circumstances that caused their breakdown.

They get told that they are 'borderline' or 'emotionally unstable' sometimes it seems *by default.*

Others develop mental *illnesses,* depression, anxiety, bipolar disorder, schizophrenia, which have biological, psychological and social causes. They do exist, for women just as they do for men, and to deny that is to gaslight the women who are suffering with them. But women need expert help from professionals who also understand what oppression is and the trauma it causes.

Sadly, that is too often lacking.

Third, we discover our mental health problems are less important because they *are* women's problems. There are insufficient services and not enough people trained to help us with them. There isn't enough awareness about the kind of mental *and* physical health problems that women, in particular, experience.

We get forgotten, discounted and written off by society.

We must demand, *and help others,* to be listened to and believed.

I began this book with nostalgia for the 1980s when it seemed that feminism really was making a difference to women's mental health. But I was reminded the feminist mental health circles I moved in then were white and middle class. There was inequality and marginalisation of those who didn't 'fit', Black women, working-class women, trans women, and severely mentally ill women.

Feminism *has* moved on from then, though is *still* at war with itself over trans rights.

However, to me, it seems as though feminist thinking about mental health has also become stuck – in its past fights with psychiatry. Some are *still* asking questions like 'Is depression "real" or an invention of "Big Pharma"?' (It is if you've had it.) 'Is there such a thing as "Premenstrual Dysphoric Disorder"?' (Ditto.) Aren't psychiatrists with their prescription pads trying to drug women into submission on behalf of the patriarchy?

Well, *no.*

There was, and still is, plenty about psychiatry to be angry about (and I say that as a psychiatrist). Diagnosing women as being 'borderline' or

EUPD is only one of those things. But as a feminist I think we should not only be challenging the *oppression* of women in our society, which is legion and contributes to so much suffering, but also be helping women to get better treatment for mental illnesses such as severe *depression* which is *real*. It *isn't* all a 'normal reaction to trauma'. Some haven't experienced any trauma and biology plays a part too.

Nevertheless, too often in mental health care the biological part of the bio-psycho-social triad of lenses through which we understand mental illness seems to dominate. There is only medication, insufficient time to talk, no access to therapy and also a focus on 'risk' to the exclusion of everything else. And mental health services also need to look through the fourth lens I described, which focuses on the powerful economic and political forces that impact negatively on women's lives – because oppression and discrimination have a massive impact on their mental health.

Addressing the consequences of oppression is sometimes dismissed as being 'too political' or just too risky for mental health professionals to get involved in, even when our own institutions are involved.

In 2023, refusal of the *British Journal of Psychiatry* to agree to the retraction of a highly controversial paper from 2011 caused a stir in the media.[2] The paper concluded that women who have had an abortion have an 81% increased risk of developing mental health problems, and was submitted as part of the evidence to overturn *Roe v. Wade* in the US Supreme court. An independent panel resigned when their advice to retract was not accepted.

Many women psychiatrists were particularly disappointed and angry about that decision. As feminists, we know that challenging the way in which flawed 'evidence' can be used to support oppression is *always* going to be viewed as a political act.

Philippa Greenfield, the new presidential co-lead for women's mental health at the Royal College of Psychiatrists, told me:

> We know the harm caused by inequality and misuse of power in our society. But we continue to fail to meaningfully act on this because solutions fundamentally mean challenging and dismantling this power dynamic.

Making a difference means bringing people with different views to work together and that means a need for openness, honesty and *sharing power*.

Philippa is determined to mainstream issues of women's mental health within the psychiatric workforce and, 'Ensure a women's lens is being brought to all we do in the Royal College.'

It's really welcome to hear her say that.

So, what we need is *much better* evidence about women's mental health and illness, which has been chronically underfunded. We want national data to be *routinely* broken down by sex and gender so that the problems faced by women are easier to identify and research. And gender-based violence should be part of the core work of mental health services. We *must* find better ways to help the women so affected by trauma that they are forced to struggle on while being re-traumatised by poor mental health care. Some only belatedly find the kind of support they really needed.

Others are no longer here.

As feminists we should be campaigning for more investment in problems such as eating disorders, which are more common in women and grossly underfunded. *So many* of the women who told me their stories in this book initially suffered from eating disorders and didn't receive adequate and timely treatment.

And most of all we should be campaigning for more humane care that puts *all* women, regardless of their race, religion, age, class, ability, sexuality and whether they identify as cis or trans women, at the *centre* of their care.

As a patient, I want to be treated with respect, kindness and compassion. I don't want someone to *tell* me they are 'trauma-informed', I want them to *act* like they are: to listen to me and take me seriously.

It's essential that I can trust them.

And I don't want to be told what to do. I want to know about different ways that I might be helped and given sufficient information to be able to make an informed choice. But I do want a professional to be honest with me – as long as they don't try to impose their views on me.

It is *my life*.

As a psychiatrist, my role has always been to try to discover what is needed to help *this woman* sitting in front of me *now*, at *this moment in time*. We should never try to impose our own ideology on anyone, and that includes our views about feminism, gender, other professionals, what we believe is the right kind of therapy, politics, religion and anything else you care to mention.

It must always begin with listening to the patient or client's story. How else can we connect?

This story began not only in Manchester in 2016 but also decades before when I was a junior doctor at the Women's Therapy Centre in London. The feminist therapists of that time then moved on to train in the traditional types of therapy, such as psychoanalysis, and the 'feminist' prefix disappeared.

But a 'feminist informed' therapist, I believe, is someone who helps a woman to rediscover her own voice. The 'different voice' that the veteran feminist psychologist Carol Gilligan described. The voice that speaks the unvarnished truth but is silenced in adolescence when girls are told that they must bury their anger, repress their honest voices and 'lose their minds' to retain their relationships and make what is called 'progress' in the world.[3]

I learned in my own therapy and helped other women to see that life doesn't have to follow that script. The older women I interviewed for this book no longer cared what other people thought. They were finally recalling their different voices – still buried within them.

As women we *can* express our own 'voices' *and* have fulfilling relationships with others too, who appreciate us for who we really are. We *can* make change to our lives.

But many of us need help to find our voice once more.

We need to find those voices to speak out. To do so doesn't mean we are 'out of our minds', it means we are finding them again.

I was on the winning side in the debate that night in Manchester.

The house, unsurprisingly given that it was voting at a Women's Week event, rejected the motion that 'Men are the losers now'.

I don't doubt many men are suffering too. I have listened to them, helped them and fought for their right to better mental health care throughout my career. As the world has always been designed around men, some are bound to complain when they believe they are losing power to which they feel entitled. Nevertheless, that doesn't mean society is now biased *against* them.

It's way past time we acknowledged what is going wrong for women's mental health.

And start to do something about it.

It's not only feminism. It's social justice.

Acknowledgements

There are so many people to thank!

First of all, Catherine Barnes from Cambridge University Press who believed in this book from reading the proposal; Lori Handelman, who steered me through the writing process with such enthusiasm for it; and Maddy Belton and Dan Smith who both provided much-needed encouragement early on in this project.

Thanks so much to everyone named below who gave me their time, told me their stories and shared their knowledge and expertise.

Alice, Andrea, Angie, Annie, Anya, Amrah, Asha, Becky, Catherine, Charlotte, Chris, Dani, Deborah, Elena, Ellie, Em, Emma, Emily Grace, Fern, Fiona, Freida, Freya, George, Hannah, Helen, Jade, Jane, Jennifer, Jenny, Jem, Jo, Julia, Jude, Keira, Lara, Lesley, Lisa, Liz, Lucy, Marie, Mal, Martina, Naina, Nessa, Nicki, Rabia, Rebecca, Sally, Sarah, @StrongestSmile, Susan, Sylvia, Ty, Valerie.

Gwen Adshead, Linda Allan, Dan Anderson, Stephen Anderson, Louis Appleby, Agnes Ayton, John Baker, Lucy Baldwin, Rachel Bannister, Richard Barnes, James Barrett, Caitlin Bernard, Hollie Berrigan, Erica Burman, Jane Callaghan, Roch Cantwell, Khatidja Chantler, Carolyn Chew-Graham, Anna Conway Morris, Dawn Edge, Luise Eichenbaum, Rebecca Farrington, Tamsin Ford, Tania Gergel, Philippa Greenfield, Lucy Grieve, Diane Goslar, Keir Harding, Ruth Ann Harpur, Annie Hickox, Julia Hose, Louise Howard, Ruth F. Hunt, Anna Hutchinson, Sameera Jahagirdar, Tulika Jha, Stella Kingett, Ute Landy, Finn Mackay, Cleo Madeleine, Raka Maitra, Francesca Moore, Jane Morris, Suryia Nayak, Bushra Nazir, Susie Orbach, Liliana Pasterska, Samantha Paxton, Merrick Pope, Dina Poursanidou, Gianetta Rands, Ruth Reed, Kirstein Rummery, Catherine Sacks Jones, Naomi Salisbury, Soma Sara, Jenny Shaw, Hannah Short, Sue

Sibbald, Hananna Siddiqui, Shubalade Smith, Jessica Southgate, Hel Spandler, Anna Sri, Francesca Stavrakopolou, Erin Stevens, Alice Vinten, Hope Virgo, Sam Warner, Jay Watts, Kathleen Wenaden and Colin Westwood.

All of your contributions were immensely valuable.

Last, but not least, many, many thanks as always to John Manton for being there throughout!

Permissions to Quote in the Text

bell hooks for an extract from *Feminism is for Everybody: Passionate Politics*, Routledge, copyright © 2015 by Gloria Watkins. Reproduced with permission of Taylor and Francis Group, LLC, a division of Informa plc, through PLS Clear.

Luise Eichenbaum and Susie Orbach for an extract from *Inside Out, Outside In: Women's Psychology, a Feminist Psychoanalytic Approach*. London, Penguin Books, 1982. Reproduced with permission of the authors.

Sheila MacLeod for an extract from *The Art of Starvation: An Adolescence Observed*, Virago Press copyright © by Sheila MacLeod. Reproduced with permission of Little, Brown, through PLS Clear.

Rachel Bannister for an extract from 'Struggling with addiction you just need a hand to hold to see you through this'. Reproduced with permission of the *British Medical Journal*.

Rachel Cooke for an extract from 'Jeremy Gavron: "My mother was a woman who looked for solutions. Suicide was a solution."' Copyright © Guardian News & Media Ltd 2023. Reproduced with permission of *The Guardian*.

Carolyn Chew-Graham and colleagues for an extract from 'South Asian women, psychological distress and self-harm: Lessons for primary care trusts', *Health & Social Care in the Community*, 2002. Reproduced with the permission of John Wiley and Sons.

Pauline Collier for an extract from *Aversion Therapy: A Personal Account*, 2023. Reproduced with permission of *The Psychologist*.

John Stoltenberg for an extract from *Andrea Dworkin was a Trans Ally*. Boston Review, 2020. Reproduced with permission of the author.

Pat Carlen for an extract from *Criminal Women, Autobiographical Accounts*. Polity, 1985. Reproduced with permission of the publisher.

Laura Abbott and colleagues for an extract from 'Pregnancy and childbirth in English prisons: Institutional ignominy and the pains of imprisonment', *Sociology of Health & Illness*, 2020. Reproduced with permission from John Wiley and Sons.

Recovery in the Bin Collective for an extract from *A Simple Guide to Avoid Receiving a Diagnosis of Personality Disorder*. Reproduced with permission from RITB.

Ruth F. Hunt for extracts from 'I was sexually assaulted on a psychiatric ward. This can't carry on', *British Medical Journal*, 2023. Reproduced with permission of *British Medical Journal* and the author.

Notes

Introduction:

Are We Out of Our Minds?

1. www.ons.gov.uk/peoplepopulationandcommunity/birthsdeathsand marriages/deaths/bulletins/suicidesintheunitedkingdom/2021regis trations (accessed 11.11.23).
2. S. Ibrahim, I.M. Hunt and M.S Rahman. Recession, recovery and suicide in mental health patients in England: Time trend analysis. *British Journal of Psychiatry*, 2019; **215**: 608–14.
3. R.C. O'Connor, K. Wetherall, S. Cleare, et al. Suicide attempts and non-suicidal self-harm: National prevalence study of young adults. *BJPsych Open*, 2018; **3**: 142–8.
4. www.mentalhealth.org.uk/explore-mental-health/publications/men tal-health-young-women-and-girls-policy-briefing (accessed 11.11.23).
5. Adult Psychiatric Morbidity Survey: Survey of Mental Health and Wellbeing, England, 2014. https://digital.nhs.uk/data-and-informa tion/publications/statistical/adult-psychiatric-morbidity-survey/adul t-psychiatric-morbidity-survey-survey-of-mental-health-and-well being-england-2014 (accessed 11.11.23).
6. Joining the Dots: The Combined Effects of Violence, Abuse and Poverty in the Lives of Women. *Agenda*, September 2016. www.agen daalliance.org/documents/120/Joining_The_Dots_Report_Executive_ Summary.pdf (accessed 11.11.23).
7. www.gov.uk/government/publications/race-disparity-audit (accessed 11.11.23).
8. www.femicidecensus.org/wp-content/uploads/2022/02/010998-2020 -Femicide-Report_V2.pdf (accessed 11.11.23).
9. Hidden Hurt: Violence, Abuse and Disadvantage in the Lives of Women. *Agenda*, 29 January 2016. www.agendaalliance.org/our-wor k/projects-and-campaigns/violence-abuse-poverty-and-multiple-dis advantage/ (accessed 11.11.23).

10.　M. Olff. Sex and gender differences in post-traumatic stress disorder: An update. *European Journal of Psychotraumatology*. 2017; **8**: 1351204.

11.　Violence against Women: An EU-Wide Survey. *European Agency for Fundamental Rights*. Luxembourg, 2014. https://fra.europa.eu/sites/default/files/fra_uploads/fra-2014-vaw-survey-main-results-apr14_en.pdf (accessed 14.2.24).

12.　P. Andre Brouillet (1857–1914) *A Clinical Lesson at the Salpêtrière* (1887).

13.　A. Hustvedt. *Medical Muses: Hysteria in Nineteenth-Century Paris*. New York: W.W. Norton, 2011.

14.　L. Appignanesi. *Mad, Bad and Sad: A History of Women and the Mind Doctors from 1800 to the Present*. London: Hachette, UK, 2011; E. Showalter. *The Female Malady: Women, Madness, and English Culture, 1830–1980*. London: Virago, 1987.

15.　b. hooks. *Feminism is for Everybody: Passionate Politics*. London: Pluto Press, 2000.

16.　www.partnersinsalford.org/media/si5leren/11-5180-mental-health-strategy_v5.pdf (accessed 14.2.24).

17.　Adult Psychiatric Morbidity Survey, 2014.

Chapter 1:

Growing up a Girl

1.　www.nytimes.com/2021/04/01/world/europe/schools-uk-rape-culture.html (accessed 11.11.23).

2.　https://plan-uk.org/media-centre/more-than-half-of-girls-have-experienced-sexual-harassment-in-a-learning-environment (accessed 11.11.23).

3.　https://digital.nhs.uk/data-and-information/publications/statistical/mental-health-of-children-and-young-people-in-england/2023-wave-4-follow-up#data-sets (accessed 31.12.23).

4.　The next will be published in 2024.

5.　S. McManus, P.E. Bebbington, R. Jenkins, et al. *Mental Health and Wellbeing in England: The Adult Psychiatric Morbidity Survey 2014*. London: NHS Digital, 2016. https://assets.publishing.service.gov.uk/media/5a802e2fe5274a2e8ab4ea71/apms-2014-full-rpt.pdf (accessed 11.11.23).

6.　C. Millard. *A History of Self-Harm in Britain: A Genealogy of Cutting and Overdosing*. London: Palgrave MacMillan, 2015.

7.　S. Plath. *The Bell Jar*. London: Faber & Faber, 1963.

8. N. Kreitman, A.E. Philip, S. Greer, et al. Parasuicide. *British Journal of Psychiatry*, **115** (1969): 746–7.

9. N. Kessel. Self-Poisoning: II. *British Medical Journal*, 2 (1965): 1336.

10. www.thetimes.co.uk/article/anne-longfield-more-teenage-girls-admitted-to-english-hospitals-for-self-harming-5cpxhpfj2 (accessed 11.11.23).

11. T. Newlove-Delgado, T. Marcheselli, T. Williams, et al. *Mental Health of Children and Young People in England, 2022 – Wave 3 Follow Up to the 2017 Survey*. London: NHS Digital. 2022. https://digital.nhs.uk/data-and-information/publications/statistical/mental-health-of-children-and-young-people-in-england/2022-follow-up-to-the-2017-survey/data-sets (accessed 11.11.23).

12. R.C. O'Connor, K. Wetherall and S. Cleare. Suicide attempts and non-suicidal self-harm: National prevalence study of young adults. *BJPsych Open*, **4** (2018): 142–8.

13. Often Overlooked: Young Women, Poverty and Self-Harm. *Agenda*, 22 May 2020. www.agendaalliance.org/our-work/projects-and-campaigns/often-overlooked/ (accessed 11.11.23).

14. S. MacDonald, C. Sampson, R. Turley, et al. Patients' experiences of emergency hospital care following self-harm: Systematic review and thematic synthesis of qualitative research. *Qualitative Health Research*, **30** (2020): 471–85.

15. www.ons.gov.uk/peoplepopulationandcommunity/birthsdeathsandmarriages/deaths/bulletins/suicidesintheunitedkingdom/2021registrations (accessed 11.11.23).

16. https://sites.manchester.ac.uk/ncish/reports/annual-report-2023/ (accessed 11.11.23).

17. C. Rodway, S.G. Tham, S. Ibrahim, et al. Suicide in children and young people in England: A consecutive case series. *The Lancet Psychiatry*, **3** (2016): 751–9.

18. C. Rodway, S.G. Tham, S. Ibrahim, et al. Children and young people who die by suicide: Childhood-related antecedents, gender differences and service contact. *BJPsych Open*, 6 (2020): e49.

19. www.rsph.org.uk/about-us/news/instagram-ranked-worst-for-young-people-s-mental-health.html (accessed 11.11.23).

20. https://digital.nhs.uk/data-and-information/publications/statistical/mental-health-of-children-and-young-people-in-england/2022-follow-up-to-the-2017-survey/data-sets (accessed 11.11.23).

21. www.theguardian.com/technology/2019/feb/07/instagram-bans-graphic-self-harm-images-after-molly-russells-death (accessed 11.11.23).

22. www.beateatingdisorders.org.uk/recovery-information/dangers-of-p ro-ana-and-pro-mia (accessed 11.11.23).

23. www.theguardian.com/education/2022/apr/28/no-girls-are-not-put- off-by-hard-maths-katharine-birbalsingh (accessed 11.11.23).

24. www.girlguiding.org.uk/globalassets/docs-and-resources/research-a nd-campaigns/girls-attitudes-survey-2023.pdf (accessed 11.11.23).

25. https://repec-cepeo.ucl.ac.uk/cepeow/cepeowp20-13.pdf (accessed 11.11.23).

26. There is no evidence of a gender difference in perfectionism, so it isn't the 'answer' but it probably plays a part in the rise in emotional problems in young people.

27. https://girlguiding.foleon.com/girls-attitudes-survey/2022-report/saf ety (accessed 11.11.23).

28. www.ons.gov.uk/peoplepopulationandcommunity/crimeandjustice/ bulletins/crimeinenglandandwales/yearendingseptember2022#do mestic-abuse-and-sexual-offences (accessed 11.11.23).

29. www.thehotline.org/resources/what-is-gaslighting/ (accessed 11.11.23).

30. M. Rosenberg and L.I. Pearlin. Social class and self-esteem among children and adults. *American Journal of Sociology*, 84 (1978): 53–77.

31. www.gov.uk/government/news/uk-children-and-adults-to-be-safer- online-as-world-leading-bill-becomes-law (accessed 11.11.23).

32. https://epi.org.uk/wp-content/uploads/2021/01/EPI-PT_Young-peo ple's-wellbeing_Jan2021.pdf (accessed 11.11.23).

33. https://epi.org.uk/publications-and-research/bullying-a-review-of-t he-evidence/ (accessed 11.11.23).

Chapter 2:

Family Life

1. www.theguardian.com/music/2021/nov/12/britney-spears-conserva torship-terminated (accessed 17.2.24).

2. www.newyorker.com/news/american-chronicles/britney-spears-con servatorship-nightmare (accessed 17.2.24).

3. www.nytimes.com/2021/06/22/arts/music/britney-spears-conserva torship.html (accessed 17.2.24).

4. A. Esterson *Sanity, Madness and the Family*. London: Routledge, 2016.

5. www.imdb.com/title/tt0068569/ (accessed 11.11.23).

6. J. Taylor. *Why Women Are Blamed for Everything: Exposing the Culture of Victim-Blaming*. London: Constable, 2020.

7. P. Bronstein. The family environment: Where gender role socialization begins. In Worell, J., Goodheart, C.D. , eds. *Handbook of girls' and women's psychological health*. Oxford, Oxford University Press. 2006, 262–71.

8. A.M. La Greca, E.R. Mackey and K.B. Miller. The interplay of physical and psychosocial development. In J. Worell and C.D. Goodheart (eds.) *Handbook of Girls' and Women's Psychological Health*. Oxford: Oxford University Press, 2006, 252–61.

9. weareagenda.org/often-overlooked/ (accessed 11.11.23).

10. S. Maji and S. Dixit. Self-silencing and women's health: A review. *International Journal of Social Psychiatry*, **65** (2019): 3–13.

11. L. Eichenbaum and S. Orbach. *Outside In, Inside Out: Women's Psychology: A Feminist Psychoanalytic Approach*. London: Penguin Books, 1982.

12. U. Owen (ed.). *Fathers, Reflections by Daughters*. London, Virago, 1994.

13. Owen, Fathers, Reflections by Daughters.

14. D. Kandiyoti. Bargaining with patriarchy. *Gender & Society*, **2** (1988): 274–90.

15. K.W. Crenshaw. *On Intersectionality: Essential Writings*. New York: New Press, 2017.

16. C. Rodway, S.G. Tham, S. Ibrahim, et al. Suicide in children and young people in England: A consecutive case series. *The Lancet Psychiatry*, **3** (2016): 751–9.

17. S. Holt, H. Buckley and S. Whelan. The impact of exposure to domestic violence on children and young people: A review of the literature. *Child Abuse & Neglect*, **32** (2008): 797–810.

18. P. Mullen, V. Walton and S. Romans-Clarkson. Impact of sexual and physical abuse on women's mental health. *The Lancet*, **331** (1988): 841–5.

19. J.M. Masson. *The Assault on Truth: Freud's Suppression of the Seduction Theory*. New York: Farrar, Straus and Giroux, 1984.

20. F. Rush. *The Best Kept Secret: Sexual Abuse of Children*. Englewood Cliffs, NJ: Prentice-Hall, 1980.

21. F. Meinck, J. Steinert, D. Sethi, et al. *Measuring and Monitoring National Prevalence of Child Maltreatment: A Practical Handbook*. Copenhagen: World Health Organisation Regional Office for Europe, 2016.

22. I.M. Engelhard, R.J. McNally and K. van Schie. Retrieving and modifying traumatic memories: Recent research relevant to three

controversies. *Current Directions in Psychological Science,* **28** (2019): 91–6.

23.   L.S. Brown and E. Burman. Feminist Responses to the False Memory Debate. *Feminism & Psychology,* **7** (1997): 7–16.

24.   S. Warner. *Understanding the Effects of Child Sexual Abuse: Feminist Revolutions in Theory, Research and Practice.* London: Routledge, 2009.

25.   www.thetimes.co.uk/article/how-ghislaine-maxwells-defence-used-false-memory-theory-to-undermine-accusers-cnrn2zkkn (accessed 11.11.23).

26.   J. Taylor. *Sexy but Psycho: How the Patriarchy Uses Women's Trauma against Them.* London: Constable, 2022.

27.   www.nytimes.com/2020/01/31/health/bonnie-burstow-dead.html (accessed 11.11.23).

28.   I. Pote, L. Doubell, L. Brims, et al. Engaging disadvantaged and vulnerable parents: An evidence review. *Early Intervention Foundation,* 2019, 1–93. www.eif.org.uk/report/engaging-disadvantaged-and-vulnerable-parents-an-evidence-review (accessed 11.11.23).

Chapter 3:

The Art of Starvation

1.   www.nytimes.com/2021/04/28/well/family/teens-eating-disorders.html (accessed 11.11.23).

2.   www.rcpsych.ac.uk/news-and-features/latest-news/detail/2022/02/10/eating-disorders-in-children-at-crisis-point-as-waiting-lists-for-routine-care-reach-record-levels?searchTerms=eating%20disorders (accessed 11.11.23).

3.   R.L Schmidt. *Little Girl Blue: The Life of Karen Carpenter.* Chicago: Chicago Review Press, 2011.

4.   D.L Franko, A. Keshaviah, K.T. Eddy, et al. A longitudinal investigation of mortality in anorexia nervosa and bulimia nervosa. *American Journal of Psychiatry,* **170** (2013): 917–25.

5.   M. Galmiche, P. Déchelotte, G. Lambert, et al. Prevalence of eating disorders over the 2000–2018 period: A systematic literature review. *The American Journal of Clinical Nutrition,* **109** (2019): 1402–13.

6.   M.M. Fichter and N. Quadflieg. Mortality in eating disorders: Results of a large prospective clinical longitudinal study. *International Journal of Eating Disorders,* **49** (2016): 391–401.

7. A. Ayton. Investment in training, evidence based treatment, and research are necessary to prevent future deaths in eating disorders. *British Medical Journal*, **371** (2020): m4689.

8. www.thetimes.co.uk/article/nhs-failures-led-to-death-of-five-anorexics-7shlks7gq (accessed 11.11.23).

9. H. Virgo. *Stand Tall Little Girl*. London: Trigger Press, 2019.

10. G. Russell. Bulimia nervosa: An ominous variant of anorexia nervosa. *Psychological Medicine*, **9** (1979): 429–48.

11. J.I. Hudson, E. Hiripi, H.G Pope Jr, et al. The prevalence and correlates of eating disorders in the National Comorbidity Survey Replication. *Biological Psychiatry*, **61** (2007): 348–58.

12. Source: Office for National Statistics.

13. https://mhanational.org/blog/7-important-facts-about-eating-disorders (accessed 11.11.23).

14. www.wsj.com/articles/facebook-knows-instagram-is-toxic-for-teen-girls-company-documents-show-11631620739 (accessed 11.11.23).

15. A.E. Becker. *Body, Self, and Society*. Philadelphia: University of Pennsylvania Press, 2013.

16. C.L. Kurth, D.D. Krahn, K. Nairn, et al. The severity of dieting and bingeing behaviors in college women: Interview validation of survey data. *Journal of Psychiatric Research*, **29** (1995): 211–25.

17. M. Lawrence and C. Lowenstein. Self starvation. *Spare Rib*, 1979, cited in S. MacLeod. *The Art of Starvation: Anorexia Observed*. London: Virago, 1987.

18. Y.A. Kadish. The role of culture in eating disorders. *British Journal of Psychotherapy*, **28** (2012): 435–53.

19. MacLeod, The Art of Starvation, 76.

20. www.nytimes.com/1996/10/06/magazine/karen-carpenter-s-second-life.html (accessed 11.11.23).

21. H. Bruch. *The Golden Cage: The Enigma of Anorexia Nervosa*. Cambridge, MA, Harvard University Press, 2001.

22. D.B. Mumford, A.M. Whitehouse and M Platts. Sociocultural correlates of eating disorders among Asian schoolgirls in Bradford. *British Journal of Psychiatry*, **158** (1991): 222–8.

23 C.M. Bulik, L. Blake and J. Austin. Genetics of eating disorders: What the clinician needs to know. *Psychiatric Clinics*, **42** (2019): 59–73.

24. C.M. Bulik, R. Flatt, A. Abbaspour, et al. Reconceptualizing anorexia nervosa. *Psychiatry and Clinical Neurosciences*, **73** (2019): 518–25.

25. H.C. Steinhausen. The outcome of anorexia nervosa in the 20th century. *American Journal of Psychiatry*, **159** (2002): 1284–93.

26. W.H. Kaye and C.M. Bulik. Treatment of patients with anorexia nervosa in the US – a crisis in care. *JAMA Psychiatry*, **78** (2021): 591–2.

27. www.scienceofeds.org/2012/07/07/residential-treatment-programs (accessed 11.11.23).

28. www.beateatingdisorders.org.uk/about-beat/policy-work/intensive-o utpatient-treatment/ (accessed 11.11.23).

29. A. Ayton and A. Ibrahim. Does UK medical education provide doctors with sufficient skills and knowledge to manage patients with eating disorders safely? *Postgraduate Medical Journal*, **94** (2018): 374–80.

30. C.G. Fairburn. *Cognitive Behavior Therapy and Eating Disorders*. New York: Guilford Press, 2008.

31. J. Downs, A. Ayton and L. Collins. Untreatable or unable to treat? Creating more effective and accessible treatment for long-standing and severe eating disorders. *The Lancet Psychiatry*, **10** (2023): 146–54.

32. www.thetimes.co.uk/article/eating-disorders-cost-the-economy-9-4b n-every-year-fvkqlq990 (accessed 11.11.23).

33. www.ombudsman.org.uk/sites/default/files/page/ACCESSIBILE%20 PDF%20-%20Anorexia%20Report.pdf (accessed 11.11.23); https://pub lications.parliament.uk/pa/cm201719/cmselect/cmpubadm/855/855 03.htm (accessed 11.11.23).

34. www.nice.org.uk/guidance/ng69 (accessed 11.11.23).

35. J. Pugh, J. Tan, T. Aziz, et al. The moral obligation to prioritize research into deep brain stimulation over brain lesioning procedures for severe enduring anorexia nervosa. *Frontiers in Psychiatry*, **9** (2018): 523.

36. www.independent.co.uk/news/uk/home-news/coroner-rules-zavar oni-died-of-natural-causes-744128.html (accessed 11.11.23).

Chapter 4:

The Costs of Fertility

1. S. Poirier. The Weir Mitchell Rest Cure: Doctor and Patients. *Women's Studies: An Interdisciplinary Journal*, **10** (1983): 15–40.

2. C.P. Gilman. Why I Wrote the Yellow Wallpaper. *Advances in Psychiatric Treatment*, **17** (2011): 265.

3. R.L. Cosslett. *The Year of the Cat*. London: Tinder Press, 2023, 108.

4. www.theguardian.com/news/2004/sep/30/guardianobituaries.health (accessed 11.11.23).

5. C. Boorse. Premenstrual syndrome and criminal responsibility. In *Premenstrual Syndrome: Ethical and Legal Implications in a Biomedical Perspective.* Boston: Springer, 1987, 81–124.

6. T. Bäckström, L. Andreen, V. Birzniece, et al. The role of hormones and hormonal treatments in premenstrual syndrome. *CNS Drugs,* 17 (2003): 325–42.

7. C.W. Skovlund, L.S. Mørch, L.V. Kessing, et al. Association of hormonal contraception with depression. *JAMA Psychiatry,* 73 (2016): 1154–62.

8. www.apa.org/monitor/oct02/pmdd (accessed 11.11.23).

9. womensmentalhealth.org/posts/etiology-premenstrual-dysphoric-disorder/ (accessed 11.11.23).

10. www.theguardian.com/society/2022/jun/02/dismissal-of-womens-health-problems-as-benign-leading-to-soaring-nhs-lists?CMP=Share_iOSApp_Other (accessed 11.11.23).

11. R.H. Bind, K. Sawyer and C. Pariante. Depression in pregnancy: Biological, clinical, and psychosocial effects. In M. Percudani, A. Bramante, V. Brenna and C. Pariante (eds.) *Key Topics in Perinatal Mental Health.* Cham, Switzerland: Springer International, 2022, 3–21.

12. www.nhs.uk/conditions/baby/support-and-services/feeling-depressed-after-childbirth/ (accessed 12.11.23).

13. R. VanderKruik, M. Barreix, D. Chou, T. Allen, et al. The global prevalence of postpartum psychosis: A systematic review. *BMC Psychiatry,* 17 (2017): 1–9.

14. https://maternalmentalhealthalliance.org/news/mbrrace-2023-suicide-still-leading-cause-maternal-death/ (accessed 12.11.23).

15. K. De Backer, C.A. Wilson, C. Dolman, et al. Rising rates of perinatal suicide. *British Medical Journal,* 381 (2023): e075414. doi: 10.1136/bmj-2023-075414.

16. www.npeu.ox.ac.uk/assets/downloads/mbrrace-uk/reports/maternal-report-2023/MBRRACE-UK_Maternal_Compiled_Report_2023.pdf (accessed 12.11.23).

17. www.bbc.co.uk/news/world-us-canada-64981965 (accessed 12.11.23).

18. M. Brown. Psychoses of the female body: The need for more psychosocial engagement. *Psychosis,* 13 (2021): 286–8.

19. L. Glover, J. Jomeen, T. Urquhart, et al. Puerperal psychosis: A qualitative study of women's experiences. *Journal of Reproductive and Infant Psychology,* 32 (2014): 254–69.

20. M. Hill. *Give Birth Like a Feminist: Your Body. Your Baby. Your Choices.* London: HarperCollins UK, 2019.

21. S. Miller, E. Abalos, M. Chamillard, et al. Beyond too little, too late and too much, too soon: A pathway towards evidence-based, respectful maternity care worldwide. *The Lancet*, **388** (2016): 2176–92.

22. K.L. Alcorn, A. O'Donovan, J.C. Patrick, et al. A prospective longitudinal study of the prevalence of post-traumatic stress disorder resulting from childbirth events. *Psychological Medicine*, **40** (2010): 1849–59.

23. www.latimes.com/opinion/op-ed/la-oe-mettler-natural-mother hood-breastfeeding-attachment-parenting-20171117-story.html (accessed 12.11.23).

24. E. Badinter. *Le Conflit. La femme et la mère*. Paris: Flammarion, 2010.

25. G. Dick-Read. *Childbirth without Fear: The Principles and Practice of Natural Childbirth*. London: Pinter & Martin, 2004.

26. www.theguardian.com/australia-news/2022/apr/07/melbourne-wo man-avoids-jail-for-killing-baby-by-laying-her-on-railway-tracks (accessed 12.11.23).

27. www.gov.uk/government/publications/final-report-of-the-ocken den-review (accessed 12.11.23).

28. www.nytimes.com/2022/07/28/us/politics/abortion-doctor-caitlin-b ernard-ohio.html (accessed 12.11.23).

29. https://veteranfeministsofamerica.org/interview-with-uta-landy/ (accessed 12.11.23).

30. L. Burns. *Larger Than an Orange*. London: Chatto & Windus, 2021.

31. N.L. Stotland and A.D. Shrestha. More evidence that abortion is not associated with increased risk of mental illness. *JAMA Psychiatry*, **75** (2018): 775–6.

32. www.nytimes.com/2022/07/01/us/abortion-abolitionists.html (accessed 12.11.23).

33. https://fivexmore.org/meet-the-team (accessed 12.11.23).

34. L. Murray and P.J. Cooper. Postpartum depression and child development. *Psychological Medicine*, **27** (1997): 253–60.

Chapter 5:

Women's Work

1. H. Gavron. *The Captive Wife: Conflicts of Housebound Mothers*. Harmondsworth: Penguin, 1973.

2. J. Gavron. *A Woman on the Edge of Time: A Son's Search for His Mother*. London: Scribe Publications, 2015.

3.   www.theguardian.com/books/2015/nov/04/a-woman-on-the-edge-o
     f-time-a-sons-search-for-his-mother-jeremy-gavron-review-biog
     raphy (accessed 12.11.23).
4.   B. Friedan. *The Feminine Mystique*. New York: W.W. Norton, 2010.
5.   W. Freeman and J.W. Watts. Psychosurgery during 1936–1946.
     Archives of Neurology & Psychiatry, **58** (1947): 417–25.
6.   E. Cleghorn. *Unwell Women: A Journey through Medicine and Myth in
     a Man-Made World*. London: Orion, 2021.
7.   A. Tone and M. Koziol. (F)ailing women in psychiatry: Lessons from
     a painful past. *CMAJ*, **190** (2018): E624–5.
8.   J.M. Ussher. *The Madness of Women: Myth and Experience*. London:
     Routledge, 2011, 88–9.
9.   P.R. Albert. Why is depression more prevalent in women? *Journal of
     Psychiatry and Neuroscience*, **40** (2015): 219–21.
10. Ussher, The Madness of Women.
11. J. Sadowsky. *The Empire of Depression: A New History*. Cambridge:
     Polity Press, 2020.
12. S. Plath. *The Bell Jar*. London: Faber & Faber, 2008.
13. K. Pugliesi. Women and mental health: Two traditions of feminist
     research. *Women & Health*, **19** (1992): 43–68.
14. M. Piccinelli and G. Wilkinson. Gender differences in depression:
     Critical review. *British Journal of Psychiatry*, **177** (2000): 486–92.
15. S.B. Patten. Are the Brown and Harris 'vulnerability factors' risk
     factors for depression? *Journal of Psychiatry and Neuroscience*, **16**
     (1991): 267.
16. b. hooks. *All about Love: New Visions*. New York: HarperCollins, 2016.
17. C.G. Jung. *Collected Works*. London: Routledge, 1973, **7**, 78.
18. For example, psychoanalysis (Freudian, Jungian), psychodynamic
     therapy, Humanistic. *Not specifically 'feminist'*.
19. https://thecommoner.org/wp-content/uploads/2019/10/04-federici
     .pdf (accessed 12.11.23).
20. B. Ehrenreich. *Nickel and Dimed: On (Not) Getting by in America*.
     New York: Metropolitan Books, 2010.
21. https://leanin.org/article/womens-workload-and-burnout (accessed
     12.11.23).
22. https://leanin.org/women-in-the-workplace-2020 (accessed 12.11.23).
23. www.who.int/publications-detail-redirect/9789240052895 (accessed
     12.11.23).
24. b. hooks. *Feminist Theory: From Margin to Center*. London: Pluto Press,
     2000.

25. www.nytimes.com/2020/12/23/opinion/coronavirus-women-feminism.html (accessed 12.11.23).

26. https://blogs.bmj.com/bmj/2020/07/24/rachel-bannister-on-struggling-with-addiction-you-just-need-a-hand-to-hold-to-see-you-through-this/ (accessed 12.11.23).

27. M. Maxwell. Women's and doctors' accounts of their experiences of depression in primary care: The influence of social and moral reasoning on patients' and doctors' decisions. *Chronic Illness*, **1** (2005): 61–71.

28. www.nice.org.uk/guidance/ng222 (accessed 12.11.23).

29. www.telegraph.co.uk/news/2022/07/07/escalating-crisis-one-eight-people-now-taking-antidepressants/ (accessed 12.11.23).

30. T. Lorenz, T. Rullo and S. Faubion. Antidepressant-induced female sexual dysfunction. *Mayo Clinic Proceedings*, **91** (2016): 1280–6.

31. E. Finch. Cash crisis forces closure of renowned Holloway women's therapy centre 2019. *Camden New Journal*, 5 June. www.islingtontribune.co.uk/article/cash-crisis-forces-closure-of-renowned-holloway-womens-therapy-centre (accessed 12.11.23).

32. J. Crispin. *Why I Am Not a Feminist: A Feminist Manifesto*. Brooklyn NY: Melville House, 2017.

33. Ussher, *The Madness of Women*, 88–9.

34. World Health Organization. *Women's Mental Health: An Evidence-Based Review*. Geneva: WHO, 2000.

Chapter 6:

Unheard, Ignored, Entrapped?

1. b. hooks. *Feminist Theory: From Margin to Center*. London: Pluto Press, 2000.

2. K.W. Crenshaw. *On Intersectionality: Essential Writings*. New York: New Press, 2017.

3. K. Christensen. 'With whom do you believe your lot is cast?' White feminists and racism. *Signs: Journal of Women in Culture and Society*, **22** (1997): 617–48.

4. L. Olufemi. *Feminism, Interrupted: Disrupting Power*. London: Pluto Press, 2020.

5. A. Light. *What Happened, Miss Simone? A Biography*. Edinburgh: Canongate, 2016.

6. D.R. Williams, J.A. Lawrence and B.A. Davis. Racism and health: Evidence and needed research. *Annual Review of Public Health*, **40** (2019): 105–25.

7. G. Kinouani. *Living While Black: The Essential Guide to Overcoming Racial Trauma.* London: Ebury, 2021.

8. M.M. Vance, J.M. Wade, M. Brandy, et al. Contextualizing Black women's mental health in the twenty-first century: Gendered racism and suicide-related behavior. *Journal of Racial and Ethnic Health Disparities,* 1 (2022): 83–92.

9. Vance et al., 'Contextualizing Black women's mental health in the twenty-first century'.

10. C.L Erving, C.S. Thomas and C. Frazier. Is the Black–white mental health paradox consistent across gender and psychiatric disorders? *American Journal of Epidemiology,* **188** (2019): 314–22.

11. R. Gater, B. Tomenson, C. Percival, et al. Persistent depressive disorders and social stress in people of Pakistani origin and white Europeans in UK. *Social Psychiatry and Psychiatric Epidemiology,* **44** (2009): 198–207.

12. www.ethnicity-facts-figures.service.gov.uk/health/mental-health/adults-experiencing-common-mental-disorders/latest (accessed 12.11.23).

13. www.ethnicity-facts-figures.service.gov.uk/health/mental-health/detentions-under-the-mental-health-act/latest (accessed 12.11.23).

14. J.A. Lewis, M.G. Williams, E.J Peppers, et al. Applying intersectionality to explore the relations between gendered racism and health among Black women. *Journal of Counseling Psychology,* **64** (2017): 475.

15. D. Edge and A. Rogers. Dealing with it: Black Caribbean women's response to adversity and psychological distress associated with pregnancy, childbirth, and early motherhood. *Social Science & Medicine,* **61** (2005): 15–25.

16. www.bitc.org.uk/wp-content/uploads/2020/03/bitc-race-report-bamewomenatwork-march2020.pdf (accessed 12.11.23).

17. www.ethnicity-facts-figures.service.gov.uk/uk-population-by-ethnicity/demographics/families-and-households/latest (accessed 12.11.23).

18. A. Rais, R. Burton and A. Rauf. A survey exploring gendered racism experienced by junior doctors working in psychiatry. *BJPsych Open,* **8** (2022): S109.

19. C. Chew-Graham, C. Bashir, K. Chantler, et al. South Asian women, psychological distress and self-harm: Lessons for primary care trusts. *Health & Social Care in the Community,* **10** (2002): 339–47.

20. N. Yuval-Davis. *Gender and Nation.* Thousand Oaks, CA: Sage, 1997.

21. L. Gask, S. Aseem, A. Waquas, et al. Isolation, feeling 'stuck' and loss of control: Understanding persistence of depression in British Pakistani women. *Journal of Affective Disorders,* **128** (2011): 49–55.

22. A. Kazimirski, P. Keogh, V. Kumari, et al. Forced Marriage. Prevalence and Service Response. National Centre for Social Research. Research Report No DCSF-RR128, 2009.

23. www.who.int/health-topics/female-genital-mutilation#tab=tab_1 (accessed 12.11.23).

24. www.unfpa.org/resources/female-genital-mutilation-fgm-frequently-asked-questions (accessed 12.11.23).

25. Olufemi, *Feminism, Interrupted.*

26. G. Greer. *The Whole Woman.* Cambridge: Black Swan, 2007.

27. Y. Alibhai-Brown. Asking the right questions. In *The Inner Lives of Troubled Young Muslims: Well-Being in the Age of Islamicist Terror and Anti-Muslim Hatred.* N.p.: BMSDemocracy, 2020.

28. H. Lewis. *Difficult Women: A History of Feminism in 11 Fights.* London: Jonathan Cape, 2020.

29. A. Lorde. *Sister Outsider: Essays and Speeches.* Berkeley, CA: Crossing Press, 2012, 138.

30. A. Lorde. Poetry Is Not a Luxury. *Chrysalis – A Magazine of Female Culture,* **3** (1977).

31. C.N. Adichie. *We Should All Be Feminists.* London: Vintage, 2014.

32. wholewomannetwork.org/2015/02/02/chimamanda-ngozi-adichies-press-statement-re-her-article-mornings-are-dark-i-cry-often-published-in-error-on-the-guardian/ (accessed 12.11.23).

33. https://mediadiversified.org/2015/05/06/the-language-of-distress-Black-womens-mental-health-and-invisibility/ (accessed 12.11.23).

34. www.nytimes.com/2021/04/30/health/psychiatry-racism-black-americans.html (accessed 12.11.23); www.rcpsych.ac.uk/news-and-features/latest-news/detail/2020/07/14/president%27s-open-letter-on-systemic-racism (accessed 12.11.23).

35. Lorde, Sister Outsider, 112.

36. www.dailymail.co.uk/news/article-11494897/Lady-Susan-Hussey-victim-remorseless-cruel-blame-culture-says-close-friend.html (accessed 12.11.23).

37. S. Fernando. *Institutional Racism in Psychiatry and Clinical Psychology.* London: Palgrave Macmillan, 2017.

38. https://southallBlacksisters.org.uk/news/sbss-victory-against-ealing-council/ (accessed 12.11.23).

39. Light, What Happened, Miss Simone?

Chapter 7:

Where Gender, Sex and Mental Health Collide

1. www.thetimes.co.uk/article/april-ashley-transgender-pioneer-qmfn63ltcsd (accessed 12.11.23).

2. R. East. The extraordinary case of top model April Ashley: Her secret is out. *The People,* 19 November 1961.

3. Lord Maugham. Why I think the judge was wrong over April. *The Sunday People*. 8 February 1970.

4. www.youtube.com/watch?v=8VRRWuryb4k (accessed 12.11.23).

5. www.nytimes.com/1973/12/23/archives/the-issue-is-subtle-the-deba te-still-on-the-apa-ruling-on.html (accessed 12.11.23).

6. H. Spandler and S. Carr. Lesbian and bisexual women's experiences of aversion therapy in England. *History of the Human Sciences*, **35** (2022): 218–36.

7. www.bps.org.uk/psychologist/aversion-therapy-personal-account (accessed 12.11.23).

8. H. Spandler and S. Carr. A history of lesbian politics and the psy professions. *Feminism & Psychology*, **31** (2021): 119–39.

9. LGBT in Britain: Health report (2018). *Stonewall*, November 2018. www .stonewall.org.uk/resources/lgbt-britain-health-2018 (accessed 27.02.24).

10. www.thetimes.co.uk/article/were-just-sexual-objects-to-men-says-m elania-geymonat-victim-of-homophobic-attack-d8ffgdst9?shareToke n=7c5ff0e4b6c817364b3f811875c8cde0 (accessed 12.11.23).

11. M. Gevisser. *The Pink Line: Journeys across the World's Queer Frontiers*. New York: Farrar, Straus and Giroux, 2020.

12. J. Morris. *Conundrum*. London: Faber & Faber, 2018.

13. S. Faye. *The Transgender Issue: An Argument for Justice*. London: Penguin, 2021.

14. LGBT in Britain: Health report (2018).

15. Faye, The Transgender Issue.

16. www.theguardian.com/society/2016/jul/10/meet-the-gender-reassign ment-surgeons-demand-is-going-through-the-roof (accessed 12.11.23).

17. www.nsun.org.uk/transitioning-out-of-psychiatry/ (accessed 12.11.23).

18. www.scotsman.com/news/opinion/columnists/scotland-should-not-deny-trans-womens-human-rights-because-of-predatory-men-vic tor-madrigal-borloz-3954832 (accessed 12.11.23).

19. www.scotsman.com/news/politics/nicola-sturgeon-urged-to-pause-gender-reform-plans-following-un-womens-safety-concerns-393414 5 (accessed 12.11.23).

20. S. Firestone. *The Dialectic of Sex: The Case for Feminist Revolution*. New York: Farrar, Straus and Giroux, 1970.

21. www.bostonreview.net/articles/john-stoltenberg-andrew-dworkin-w as-trans-ally/ (accessed 12.11.23).

22. https://signsjournal.org/exploring-transgender-law-and-politics/ (accessed 12.11.23).

23. H. Joyce. *Trans: Where Ideology Meets Reality*. London: Oneworld, 2021.

24. https://cass.independent-review.uk (accessed 12.11.23).

25. A.L. De Vries, J.K. McGuire and T.D. Steensma. Young adult psychological outcome after puberty suppression and gender reassignment. *Pediatrics*, **134** (2014): 696–704.

26. www.nytimes.com/2022/09/26/health/top-surgery-transgender-teen agers.html (accessed 12.11.23).

27. L. Littman. Parent reports of adolescents and young adults perceived to show signs of a rapid onset of gender dysphoria. *PLoS One*, **13** (2018): e0202330.

28. www.theguardian.com/lifeandstyle/2021/oct/05/finn-mackay-the-wr iter-hoping-to-help-end-the-gender-wars (accessed 12.11.23).

29. F. Mackay. *Female Masculinities and the Gender Wars: The Politics of Sex*. London: Bloomsbury, 2021.

30. https://slate.com/human-interest/2020/06/jk-rowling-trans-men-ter f.html (accessed 12.11.23).

31. womansplaceuk.org/2020/02/17/the-natal-female-question/ (accessed 12.11.23).

32. J. Cohn. Some limitations of 'Challenges in the care of transgender and gender-diverse youth: An endocrinologist's view'. *Journal of Sex & Marital Therapy*, **49** (2023): 599–615.

33. https://psychiatry.duke.edu/blog/gender-dysphoria-and-eating-dis orders (accessed 12.11.23).

34. www.bbc.co.uk/news/uk-65860272 (accessed 12.11.23).

35. Mackay, Female Masculinities and the Gender Wars.

36. www.rcpsych.ac.uk/pdf/PS02_18.pdf (accessed 12.11.23).

37. *The Extraordinary Life of April Ashley*, Channel 4 television.

Chapter 8:

Survivors of Male Violence

1. E. Pizzey and A. Forbes. *Scream Quietly or the Neighbours Will Hear*. Harmondsworth: Penguin, 1974.

2. www.theguardian.com/society/2023/jun/18/women-forced-to-retur n-to-violent-homes-as-shortage-of-uk-refuge-places-leads-to-crisis (accessed 12.11.23).

3. H. Kennedy. *Eve Was Framed: Women and British Justice*. London: Vintage, 2011.

4. www.who.int/news-room/fact-sheets/detail/violence-against-wome n (accessed 12.11.23).

5. M. Wallace, V. Gillispie-Bell, K. Cruz, et al. Homicide during pregnancy and the postpartum period in the United States, 2018–2019. *Obstetrics and Gynecology*, **138** (2021): 762.

6. https://aifs.gov.au/sites/default/files/publication-documents/ressu m1_0.pdf (accessed 12.11.23).

7. S. Oram, H.L. Fisher, H. Minnis, et al. The Lancet Psychiatry Commission on intimate partner violence and mental health: Advancing mental health services, research, and policy. *The Lancet Psychiatry*, **9** (2022): 487–524.

8. J. Taylor. *Sexy but Psycho: How the Patriarchy Uses Women's Trauma against Them*. London: Constable, 2022.

9. https://theconversation.com/why-victims-of-domestic-abuse-dont-l eave-four-experts-explain-176212 (accessed 12.11.23).

10. S. Walby and J. Allen. *Domestic Violence, Sexual Assault and Stalking: Findings from the British Crime Survey*. London: Home Office, 2004.

11. H. Lewis. *Difficult Women: A History of Feminism in 11 Fights*. London: Jonathan Cape, 2020.

12. www.theduluthmodel.org/what-is-the-duluth-model/ (accessed 12.11.23).

13. www.thetimes.co.uk/article/why-i-have-spent-a-decade-counting-m urdered-women-qwg0thszv (accessed 12.11.23).

14. www.femicidecensus.org/data-matters-every-woman-matters/#_ftnr ef1 (accessed 12.11.23).

15. S. Walby. *The Cost of Domestic Violence*. London: Women and Equality Unit (DTI), 2004.

16. www.theguardian.com/society/2022/feb/27/suicide-by-domestic-violence-call-to-count-the-hidden-toll-of-womens-lives (accessed 12.11.23).

17. A. Kazimirski, P. Keogh, V. Kumari, et al. Forced Marriage. Prevalence and Service Response. Research Report No DCSF-RR128. London: National Centre for Social Research, 2009.

18. www.gov.uk/government/publications/application-for-benefits-for-v isa-holder-domestic-violence (accessed 12.11.23).

19. www.theguardian.com/uk-news/2022/jun/22/honour-killings-dev ils-work-bekhal-banaz-mahmod (accessed 12.11.23).

20. S. Flynn, L. Gask, L. Appleby, et al. Homicide–suicide and the role of mental disorder: A national consecutive case series. *Social Psychiatry and Psychiatric Epidemiology*, **51** (2016): 877–84.

21. S. Flynn, L. Gask and J. Shaw. Newspaper reporting of homicide-suicide and mental illness. *BJPsych bulletin*, **39** (2015): 268–72.

22. C.A. Lee. *A Fine Day for a Hanging: The Real Ruth Ellis Story*. London: Mainstream Publishing, 2012.

23. H. Kennedy. *Misjustice: How British Law is Failing Women*. London: Vintage, 2019.

24. https://hansard.parliament.uk/Commons/1994-05-17/debates/f1 e14017-f874-416c-8a08-2ad7ccffbd25/Homicide(DefenceOfProvocati on) (accessed 12.11.23).

25. www.bbc.co.uk/news/uk-47724697 (accessed 12.11.23).

26. Kennedy, *Misjustice*.

27. M. Olff. Sex and gender differences in post-traumatic stress disorder: An update. *European Journal of Psychotraumatology*, **8** (2017): 1351204.

28. www.theguardian.com/society/2023/jan/20/home-office-vows-to-act-over-invasive-personal-record-requests-in-cases (accessed 12.11.23).

29. www.independent.co.uk/life-style/health-and-families/amber-heard-borderline-personality-disorder-b2068992.html (accessed 12.11.23).

30. www.telegraph.co.uk/news/2023/01/14/female-soldiers-raped-col leagues-misdiagnosed-personality-disorder/ (accessed 12.11.23).

31. L. Perry. *The Case against the Sexual Revolution*. Cambridge: Polity, 2022.

32. L. Finlayson, L. *An Introduction to Feminism*. Cambridge: Cambridge University Press, 2016.

33. www.gov.uk/government/publications/police-super-complaints-forc e-response-to-police-perpetrated-domestic-abuse/police-perpet rated-domestic-abuse-report-on-the-centre-for-womens-justice-sup er-complaint (accessed 12.11.23).

34. https://police-me-too.co.uk (accessed 12.11.23).

35. www.theguardian.com/commentisfree/2022/feb/02/i-recognise-only-to o-well-the-horror-stories-of-misogyny-in-the-met (accessed 12.11.23).

36. www.womensaid.org.uk/information-support/the-survivors-hand book/im-worried-about-someone-else/ (accessed 12.11.23); www.psy com.net/help-friend-sexually-assaulted-dos-donts (accessed 12.11.23).

Chapter 9:

Locked Away

1. J. O'Dwyer and P. Carlen. Josie: Surviving Holloway ... and Other Women's Prisons. In P. Carlen et al. (eds.) *Criminal Women: Autobiographical Accounts*. Cambridge: Polity, 1985, 138–81.

2. J. Corston. *The Corston Report: A Review of Women with Particular Vulnerabilities in the Criminal Justice System.* London: Home Office, 2007. www.asdan.org.uk/media/ek3p22qw/corston-report-march-2007.pdf (accessed 12.11.23).

3. https://assets.publishing.service.gov.uk/government/uploads/system/uploads/attachment_data/file/1119965/statistics-on-women-and-the-criminal-justice-system-2021-.pdf (accessed 12.11.23).

4. www.ons.gov.uk/peoplepopulationandcommunity/crimeandjustice/articles/homicideinenglandandwales/march2022#suspects-in-homicide-cases (accessed 12.11.23).

5. www.prisonpolicy.org/reports/pie2023women.html (accessed 12.11.23).

6. www.prisonstudies.org/sites/default/files/resources/downloads/world_female_imprisonment_list_5th_edition.pdf (accessed 12.11.23).

7. www.nytimes.com/2019/11/08/us/tondalao-hall-oklahoma-commutation.html (accessed 12.11.23).

8. https://publications.parliament.uk/pa/cm5803/cmselect/cmjust/265/report.html (accessed 12.11.23).

9. C. Smart. *Women, Crime and Criminology (Routledge Revivals): A Feminist Critique.* London: Routledge, 2013.

10. C.A. Lee. *One of Your Own: The Life and Death of Myra Hindley.* London: Mainstream Publishing, 2011.

11. N. Singleton, R. Gatward and H. Meltzer. *Psychiatric Morbidity among Prisoners in England and Wales.* London: Stationery Office, 1998.

12. K. Hawton, L. Linsell, T. Adeniji, et al. Self-harm in prisons in England and Wales: An epidemiological study of prevalence, risk factors, clustering, and subsequent suicide. *The Lancet,* **383** (2014): 1147–54.

13. S. Campbell. *Breakfast at Bronzefield.* London: Sophie Campbell Books, 2020.

14. www.centreformentalhealth.org.uk/publications/prison-mental-health-services-england-2023/ (accessed 12.11.23).

15. L. Baldwin, M. Elwood and C. Brown. Criminal Mothers: The Persisting Pains of Maternal Imprisonment. In G. Grace, M. O'Neill, T. Walker, et al. *Criminal Women: Gender Matters.* Bristol: Bristol University Press, 2022, 107–31.

16. L. Baldwin. Motherhood disrupted: Reflections of post-prison mothers. *Emotion, Space and Society,* **26** (2018): 49–56.

17. L. Baldwin. *Motherhood in and after Prison. The Impact of Maternal Incarceration.* Hook, Hampshire: Waterside Press, 2022.

18. L. Abbott, T. Scott and H. Thomas. Pregnancy and childbirth in English prisons: Institutional ignominy and the pains of imprisonment. *Sociology of Health & Illness*, **42** (2020): 660–75.

19. L. Abbott, T. Scott and H. Thomas. Compulsory separation of women prisoners from their babies following childbirth: Uncertainty, loss and disenfranchised grief. *Sociology of Health & Illness*, **45** (2023): 971–88.

20. www.bbc.co.uk/news/uk-england-37734706 (accessed 12.11.23).

21. S. Fazel, T. Ramesh and K. Hawton. Suicide in prisons: An international study of prevalence and contributory factors. *The Lancet Psychiatry* **4** (2017): 946–52.

22. www.inquest.org.uk/2019-update-still-dying (accessed 12.11.23).

23. G. Adshead and E. Horne. *The Devil You Know: Encounters in Forensic Psychiatry*. London: Faber & Faber, 2021.

24. G. Adshead. Same but different: Constructions of female violence in forensic mental health. *IJFAB: International Journal of Feminist Approaches to Bioethics*, **4** (2011): 41–68.

25. S. Ali and G. Adshead. Just like a woman: Gender role stereotypes in forensic psychiatry. *Frontiers in Psychiatry*, 13 (2022): 840837.

26. www.inquest.org.uk/deaths-in-custody-a-form-of-violence-against-women (accessed 12.11.23).

27. www.crimeandjustice.org.uk/sites/crimeandjustice.org.uk/files/PSJ%20255%20July%202021.pdf (accessed 12.11.23); *Mental Health Nursing*. Special Issue: Criminal Justice and Mental Health. April 2023.

28. www.crimeandjustice.org.uk/resources/trauma-informed-prisons-paradox-or-paradigm (accessed 12.11.23).

29. https://prisonreformtrust.org.uk/blog-welcome-steps-towards-a-women-centred-approach/ (accessed 12.11.23).

30. www.gov.uk/government/news/location-of-first-ground-breaking-residential-women-s-centre-revealed (accessed 12.11.23).

31. www.womenatwish.org.uk (accessed 12.11.23); womeninprison.org.uk/support/womens-centres (accessed 12.11.23).

Chapter 10:

Borderline

1. K. Badman. *The Final Years of Marilyn Monroe: The True Story*. Dover, DE: Quarto Publishing Group, 2012.

2. M. Monroe. *Fragments: Poems, Intimate Notes, Letters*. New York: Farrar, Straus and Giroux, 2010.

3. M.H. Stone. Long-term outcome in personality disorders. *British Journal of Psychiatry*, **162** (1993): 299–313.

4. American Psychiatric Publishing. *Diagnostic and Statistical Manual of Mental Disorders: DSM-5* (5th ed.). Washington, DC: APP, 2013.

5. J. Corston. *The Corston Report: A Review of Women with Particular Vulnerabilities in the Criminal Justice System*. London: Home Office, 2007. www.asdan.org.uk/media/ek3p22qw/corston-report-march-2007.pdf (accessed 12.11.23).

6. www.psychiatry.org/psychiatrists/practice/dsm (accessed 12.11.23).

7. www.beamconsultancy.co.uk/the-blog/2020/12/18/borderline-personality-disorder-and-being-ill (accessed 12.11.23).

8. S. Schiff. *The Witches: Salem, 1692*. New York: Little Brown, 2015.

9. M. Doyle, D. While, P.L. Mok, et al. Suicide risk in primary care patients diagnosed with a personality disorder: A nested case control study. *BMC Family Practice*, **17** (2016): 1–9.

10. https://sites.manchester.ac.uk/ncish/reports/annual-report-2023/ (accessed 12.11.23).

11. http://documents.manchester.ac.uk/display.aspx?DocID=37564 (accessed 12.11.23).

12. https://recoveryinthebindotorg.files.wordpress.com/2016/02/ritb-how-not-to-get-a-diagnosis-of-pd-guide.pdf (accessed 12.11.23).

13. G. Lewis and L. Appleby. Personality disorder: The patients psychiatrists dislike. *British Journal of Psychiatry*, **153** (1988): 44–9.

14. P. Tyrer. Threading a pathway through the forest of mood and personality disorders: Commentary on … Bordering on the bipolar. *BJPsych Advances*, **26** (2020): 58–60.

15. www.rcpsych.ac.uk/docs/default-source/improving-care/better-mh-policy/position-statements/ps01_20.pdf?sfvrsn=85af7fbc_2 (accessed 12.11.23).

16. www.wnyc.org/story/53922-borderline-personality-disorder (accessed 12.11.23).

17. G.E. Vaillant. The beginning of wisdom is never calling a patient a borderline; or the clinical management of immature defenses in the treatment of individuals with personality disorders. *The Journal of Psychotherapy Practice and Research*, **1** (1992): 117.

18. R. Dodds. Borderline personality disorder: My greatest asset. *The Lancet Psychiatry*, **8** (2021): 188–90.

19. J.L. Herman. *Trauma and Recovery: From Domestic Abuse to Political Terror.* New York: HarperCollins, 1992.

20. D. Orr. *Motherwell: A Girlhood.* London: Weidenfeld & Nicolson, 2020.

21. www.theguardian.com/commentisfree/2017/sep/23/afford-private-mental-health-treatment (accessed 12.11.23).

22. There was insufficient published scientific evidence of their effectiveness which meant therapeutic communities were not recommended by NICE in 2015. National Collaborating Centre for Mental Health. Borderline personality disorder: Treatment and management. Leicester: British Psychological Society, 2009. https://pubmed.ncbi.nlm.nih.gov/21796831/ (accessed 12.11.23).

23. P. Hyde. Report to Congress on Borderline personality Disorder. Pub. no. 4644. Substance Abuse and Mental Health Service Administration, 2011. www.bpdcommunity.com.au/static/uploads/files/2010-report-to-congress-on-bpd-wfcoawcbhzjd.pdf (accessed 12.11.23).

24. National Confidential Inquiry into Suicide and Safety in Mental Health. *Safer Care for Patients with Personality Disorder.* Manchester: NCISH, 2018.

25. L. Dimeff and M.M. Linehan. Dialectical behavior therapy in a nutshell. *The California Psychologist,* **34** (2001): 10–13.

26. Mentalisation-based therapy is also recommended by NICE guidance but is less commonly available.

27. www.selfinjurysupport.org.uk (accessed 12.11.23).

28. www.bbc.co.uk/news/uk-england-gloucestershire-64490848.amp (accessed 12.11.23).

29. https://stopsim.co.uk (accessed 12.11.23).

30. www.england.nhs.uk/long-read/nhs-england-position-on-serenity-integrated-mentoring-and-similar-models/ (accessed 12.11.23).

31. https://stopsim.co.uk (accessed 12.11.23).

32. www.mentalcapacitylawandpolicy.org.uk/suicide-and-the-misuse-of-capacity-in-conversation-with-dr-chloe-beale/ (accessed 12.11.23).

33. www.nice.org.uk/guidance/cg78 (accessed 12.11.23).

34. P. Luyten, C. Campbell and P. Fonagy. Rethinking the relationship between attachment and personality disorder. *Current Opinion in Psychology,* **37** (2021): 109–13.

35. C. Shaw and G. Proctor. Women at the margins: A critique of the diagnosis of borderline personality disorder. *Feminism & Psychology,* **15** (2005): 483–90.

Chapter 11:

Failed by Mental Health Care

1. C. Hilton. A woman the government feared: Barbara Robb. In G. Rands (ed.) *Women's Voices in Psychiatry: A Collection of Essays.* Oxford: Oxford University Press, 2018, 205.
2. B. Robb. *Sans Everything: A Case to Answer.* Edinburgh: Nelson, 1967.
3. https://digital.library.upenn.edu/women/bly/madhouse/madhouse .html (accessed 12.11.23).
4. I.E. Sommer and L.E. DeLisi. Precision psychiatry and the clinical care for people with schizophrenia: Sex, race and ethnicity in relation to social determinants of mental health. *Current Opinion in Psychiatry,* **35** (2022): 137–9.
5. www.york.ac.uk/media/healthsciences/images/research/prepare/re portsandtheircoverimages/Womens%20Priorities%20for%20Womens %20Health%20-%20summary2.pdf (accessed 12.11.23).
6. https://assets.publishing.service.gov.uk/government/uploads/sys tem/uploads/attachment_data/file/765821/The_Womens_Mental_H ealth_Taskforce_-_final_report1.pdf (accessed 12.11.23).
7. S. Smith. Gender differences in antipsychotic prescribing. *International Review of Psychiatry,* **22** (2010): 472–84.
8. A. Steinberg. Prone restraint cardiac arrest: A comprehensive review of the scientific literature and an explanation of the physiology. *Medicine, Science and the Law,* **61** (2021): 215–26.
9. T. Meehan, M. McGovern, D. Keniry, et al. Living with restraint: Reactions of nurses and lived experience workers to restrictions placed on the use of prone restraint. *International Journal of Mental Health Nursing,* **31** (2022): 888–96.
10. R. Gallop, E. McCay, M. Guha, et al. The experience of hospitalization and restraint of women who have a history of childhood sexual abuse. *Health Care for Women International,* **20** (1999): 401–16.
11. A. Walters. Girls with ADHD: Underdiagnosed and untreated. *The Brown University Child and Adolescent Behavior Letter,* **34** (2018): 8.
12. L. Hull, K.V. Petrides and W. Mandy. The female autism phenotype and camouflaging: A narrative review. *Journal of Autism and Developmental Disorders,* **7** (2020): 306–17.
13. J. Hook and D. Devereux. Sexual boundary violations: Victims, perpetrators and risk reduction. *BJPsych Advances,* **24** (2018): 374–83.
14. P. Chesler. *Women and Madness.* Chicago: Chicago Review Press, 2018.

15. T. Garrett and J.D. Davis. The prevalence of sexual contact between British clinical psychologists and their patients. *Clinical Psychology and Psychotherapy*, **5** (1998): 253–63.

16. K.S. Pope. *Sexual Involvement with Therapists: Patient Assessment, Subsequent Therapy, Forensics.* Washington, DC: American Psychological Association, 1994.

17. www.theguardian.com/uk/1999/jun/13/theobserver.uknews1?CMP= Share_iOSApp_Other (accessed 12.11.23); www.dailymail.co.uk/fema il/article-1035830/He-stroke-A-victim-male-nurse-preyed-anorexic-g irls-tells-story.html (accessed 12.11.23).

18. www.verita.net/wp-content/uploads/2022/06/An-independent-inves tigation-into-the-conduct-of-David-Britten-at-the-Peter-Dally-clinic- 1.pdf (accessed 12.11.23).

19. D. Veale, E. Robins, A.B. Thomson, et al. No safety without emotional safety. *The Lancet Psychiatry*, **10** (2023): 65–70.

20. www.leedsandyorkpft.nhs.uk/news/wp-content/uploads/sites/4/2022/0 2/Updated-Sexual-Safety-A5-8pp-Leaflet.170622.pdf (accessed 12.11.23).

21. www.theguardian.com/society/2023/may/23/nhs-england-mental-he alth-trusts-record-26000-sexual-abuse-incidents (accessed 12.11.23).

22. M. Foley and I. Cummins. Reporting sexual violence on mental health wards. *The Journal of Adult Protection*, **20** (2018): 93–100.

23. www.bmj.com/content/381/bmj.p1105/rr-0 (accessed 12.11.23).

24. www.cqc.org.uk/sites/default/files/20180911c_sexualsafetymh_re port.pdf (accessed 12.11.23).

25. A.R. Singh. Are women's mental health units needed? In G. Rands (ed.) *Women's Voices in Psychiatry: A Collection of Essays.* Oxford: Oxford University Press, 2018.

26. www.mentalhealthtoday.co.uk/blog/crisis-care/can-we-aim-higher-t han-single-sex-mental-health-wards (accessed 12.11.23).

27. K. Abel and S. Rees. Reproductive and sexual health of women service users: What's the fuss? Commentary on . . . addressing the sexual and reproductive health needs of women who use mental health services. *Advances in Psychiatric Treatment*, **16** (2010): 279–80.

28. H. Hope, M. Pierce, E.D. Johnstone, et al. The sexual and reproductive health of women with mental illness: A primary care registry study. *Archives of Women's Mental Health*, **25** (2022): 585–93.

29. Known on twitter as @DrEm_79.

30. www.independent.co.uk/news/health/mental-health-abuse-chil dren-huntercombe-b2270448.html# (accessed 12.11.23).

31. www.dailymail.co.uk/news/article-11896133/Police-investigated-24-ca ses-reported-rape-18-sexual-assault-Kent-psychiatric-hospital.html (accessed 12.11.23).

32. www.bbc.co.uk/news/uk-england-manchester-64318583 (accessed 12.11.23); www.thetimes.co.uk/article/west-lane-hospital-inquiries-identify-119-failures-over-deaths-of-three-teenage-girls-at-nhs-trus t-qgf2fbjx2 (accessed 12.11.23).

33. www.bbc.co.uk/programmes/m001ckxr (accessed 12.11.23).

34. Chesler, Women and Madness.

35. S. Warner. *Understanding the Effects of Child Sexual Abuse: Feminist Revolutions in Theory, Research and Practice.* London: Routledge, 2009.

36. G. Rands (ed.). *Women's Voices in Psychiatry: A Collection of Essays.* Oxford: Oxford University Press, 2018.

37. www.mind.org.uk/information-support/guides-to-support-and-ser vices/advocacy/what-is-advocacy/ (accessed 12.11.23).

38. Hilton, 'A woman the government feared: Barbara Robb', 214.

Chapter 12:

Written Off Too Soon

1. M. Attwood. *The Handmaid's Tale.* Toronto, Ont: McCleland & Stewart, 1985.

2. www.ala.org/advocacy/bbooks/frequentlychallengedbooks/top10 (accessed 12.11.23).

3. www.newstatesman.com/politics/2013/04/margaret-thatcher-femin ist-icon (accessed 12.11.23).

4. www.margaretthatcher.org/document/103811 (accessed 12.11.23).

5. www.telegraph.co.uk/news/picturegalleries/celebritynews/9223149/ Mary-Beard-hits-back-at-AA-Gill-after-he-brands-her-too-ugly-for-te levision.html (accessed 12.11.23).

6. V. Smith. *Hags: The Demonisation of Middle-Aged Women.* London: Fleet, 2023.

7. www.gov.uk/government/news/landmark-survey-seeks-womens-vie ws-on-reproductive-health (accessed 12.11.23).

8. www.bipolaruk.org/blog/bipolar-uk-evidence-to-inform-womens-he alth-strategy (accessed 12.11.23).

9. M. Leonhardt. Low mood and depressive symptoms during perimenopause: Should General Practitioners prescribe hormone

replacement therapy or antidepressants as the first-line treatment? *Post Reproductive Health*, **25** (2019): 124–30.

10. S. Orgad and C. Rottenberg. Mediating menopause: Feminism, neoliberalism, and biomedicalisation. *Feminist Theory*, **13** (2023): 14647001231182030.

11. www.nytimes.com/2021/05/25/opinion/feminist-menopause.html (accessed 12.11.23).

12. www.carersuk.org/policy-and-research/key-facts-and-figures/ (accessed 12.11.23).

13. www.womenshealth.gov/a-z-topics/caregiver-stress#references (accessed 12.11.23).

14. M. Fitting, P. Rabins, M.J. Lucas, et al. Caregivers for dementia patients: A comparison of husbands and wives. *The Gerontologist*, **26** (1986): 248–52.

15. www.nytimes.com/2021/03/16/us/caregiving-burnout.html (accessed 12.11.23).

16. www.ons.gov.uk/peoplepopulationandcommunity/birthsdeathsand marriages/ageing/articles/profileoftheolderpopulationlivinginenglan dandwalesin2021andchangessince2011/2023-04-03#legal-partner ships (accessed 12.11.23).

17. C. Gilligan. *In a Different Voice: Psychological Theory and Women's Development*. Cambridge, MA: Harvard University Press, 1993.

18. J. Domènech-Abella, E. Lara, M. Rubio-Valera, et al. Loneliness and depression in the elderly: The role of social network. *Social Psychiatry and Psychiatric Epidemiology*, **52** (2017): 381–90.

19. www.ons.gov.uk/peoplepopulationandcommunity/birthsdeathsand marriages/deaths/bulletins/suicidesintheunitedkingdom/2022regis trations#suicide-patterns-by-age (accessed 31.12.23).

20. www.cdc.gov/nchs/data/databriefs/db464.pdf (accessed 12.11.23).

21. A. Case and A. Deaton. *Deaths of Despair and the Future of Capitalism*. Princeton, NJ: Princeton University Press, 2020.

22. B. Burstow. Understanding and ending ECT: A feminist imperative. *Canadian Woman Studies/les cahiers de la femme*, **25** (2006): 115–22.

23. www.mind.org.uk/information-support/drugs-and-treatments/elec troconvulsive-therapy-ect/ (accessed 12.11.23).

24. www.rcpsych.ac.uk/mental-health/treatments-and-wellbeing/ect (accessed 12.11.23).

25. T. Gergel. 'Shock tactics', ethics and fear: An academic and personal perspective on the case against electroconvulsive therapy. *British Journal of Psychiatry*, **220** (2022): 109–12.

26. www.independent.co.uk/news/health/electroconvulsive-therapy-bra in-mental-health-b2095155.html (accessed 12.11.23).

27. G. Kirov, S. Jauhar, P. Sienaert, et al. Electroconvulsive therapy for depression: 80 years of progress. *British Journal of Psychiatry*, **219** (2021): 594–7.

28. www.nice.org.uk/guidance/ng222/chapter/Recommendations#electr oconvulsive-therapy-for-depression (accessed 12.11.23).

29. www.mind.org.uk/information-support/drugs-and-treatments/elec troconvulsive-therapy-ect/ (accessed 12.11.23).

30. www.nhs.uk/conditions/fibromyalgia/ (accessed 12.11.23).

31. L.A. Saraswati. *Scarred: A Feminist Journey through Pain.* New York: New York University Press, 2023.

32. W. Brown *States of Injury: Power and Freedom in Late Modernity.* Princeton, NJ: Princeton University Press, 2020.

33. www.alzheimers.org.uk/about-dementia/types-dementia (accessed 12.11.23).

34. J. Chung, A. Das, X. Sun, et al. Genome-wide association and multi-omics studies identify MGMT as a novel risk gene for Alzheimer's disease among women. *Alzheimer's & Dementia*, **19** (2023): 896–908.

35. www.alzheimers.org.uk/about-us/policy-and-influencing/our-pos ition-key-dementia-challenges/dementia-research (accessed 12.11.23).

36. https://dementiastatistics.org/about-dementia/ (accessed 12.11.23).

37. www.dailymail.co.uk/news/article-1048853/Baroness-Thatcher-con stantly-repeats-forgets-husband-Denis-dead-says-daughter-Carol.ht ml (accessed 12.11.23).

38. R. Klein and S. Hawthorne. *Not Dead Yet: Feminism, Passion and Women's Liberation.* North Geelong, Vic: Spinifex Press, 2021.

39. www.gov.uk/government/publications/womens-health-strategy-for-england/womens-health-strategy-for-england (accessed 12.11.23).

40. https://ageing-better.org.uk/news/image-library-contributions-invis ible-older-women-work (accessed 12.11.23).

41. https://ethicsofcare.org/carol-gilligan/ (accessed 12.11.23).

42. www.cipd.org/uk/knowledge/guides/carer-friendly-workplace/ (accessed 12.11.23).

43. www.carersuk.org/media/chxfyc30/carers-uk-039-s-evidence-wome n-039-s-budget-group-commission-transformative-policy.pdf (accessed 12.11.23).

44. S. Faludi. American Electra: Feminism's ritual matricide. *Harper's Magazine*, **321** (2010): 29–42.

45. R.L. Jones. Imagining feminist old age: Moving beyond 'successful' ageing? *Journal of Aging Studies*, **63** (2022): 100950.

46. www.alzheimers.org.uk/about-dementia/risk-factors-and-preven tion/how-reduce-your-risk-alzheimers-and-other-dementias#5 (accessed 12.11.23).

47. M. Attwood. *The Testaments*. Toronto, Ont: McLeland and Stewart, 2019.

Conclusion

1. https://msmagazine.com/2023/09/13/texas-abortion-travel-ban-sanc tuary-city/ (accessed 12.11.23).

2. www.bbc.co.uk/news/uk-66249015 (accessed 12.11.23).

3. C. Gilligan. *Joining the Resistance*. Cambridge: Polity Press, 2013.

Index